PLEXUS - Vagus Nerve Exposed - Practical Guide

The Practical Guide To Stimulate Vagus Nerve, to Restore it and Making Sure To Keep it Healthy

A Book written by Loren Allen in collaboration with Dr. Vishen R. Kohler

© Copyright 2022 by Loren Allen - All rights reserved.

The following Book is reproduced below with the goal of providing information that is as accurate and reliable as possible. Regardless, purchasing this Book can be seen as consent to the fact that both the publisher and the author of this book are in no way experts on the topics discussed within and that any recommendations or suggestions that are made herein are for entertainment purposes only. Professionals should be consulted as needed prior to undertaking any of the action endorsed herein.

This declaration is deemed fair and valid by both the American Bar Association and the Committee of Publishers Association and is legally binding throughout the United States.

Furthermore, the transmission, duplication, or reproduction of any of the following work including specific information will be considered an illegal act irrespective of if it is done electronically or in print. This extends to creating a secondary or tertiary copy of the work or a recorded copy and is only allowed with the express written consent from the Publisher. All additional right reserved.

The information in the following pages is broadly considered a truthful and accurate account of facts and as such, any inattention, use, or misuse of the information in question by the reader will render any resulting actions solely under their purview. There are no scenarios in which the publisher or the original author of this work can be in any fashion deemed liable for any hardship or damages that may befall them after undertaking information described herein.

Table Of Contents

What is Vagus Nerve?	2
Anatomical Course	5
What does the vagus nerve affect?	12
Functions of the Vagus Nerve	14
The Role of Vagus in the Autonomic Nervous System	20
What Happens If The Vagus Nerve Is Damaged?	31
Communication Effects of Vagus Nerve Damage	34
The Functions of the Nervous System	49
How to know if your Vagus nerve is injured or compressed	56
Controlling Epilepsy: Vagus Nerve Stimulation	68
Turning Your Vagus On	80
Testing Vagus nerve activity	83
Causes of Vagus Nerve Damage	92
Vagus Nerve Stimulation	105
Who Can Benefit From This Stimulation	108

Evaluation	108
Procedure	109
Vagus Nerve Stimulation Techniques - Probiotics	**112**
What are probiotics?	114
Advantages of Taking Probiotics	120
Probiotics and Vaginal Health	123
Probiotic Supplements	124
CONCLUSION	125
Healthy Recipes for Vagus Nerve	**128**
Chili-lime Cucumber, Jicama, & Apple Sticks	**128**
Sardine Meatballs	**129**
Homemade Salsa	**130**
Kale Chips	**132**
Feta Tomato Sea Bass	**133**
Crab Stew	**134**
Trail Mix	**136**
Berry & Veggie Gazpacho	**136**
Meat-filled Phyllo (samboosek)	**138**
Raw Turmeric Cashew Nut & Coconut Balls	**140**
Ginger Tahini Dip With Veggies	**141**

Crunchy Veggie Chips	**142**
Honey Garlic Shrimp	**142**
Pita Chips	**144**
Leeks And Calamari Mix	**145**
Cucumber Rolls	**146**
Parmesan Chips	**147**
Grape, Celery & Parsley Reviver	**148**
Tomato Triangles	**149**
Asparagus Frittata	**150**
Salmon And Broccoli	**151**
Chili Mango And Watermelon Salsa	**152**
Chia Crackers	**153**
Pepper Salmon Skewers	**155**
Garlic Mussels	**157**
Superfood Spiced Apricot-sesame Bliss Balls	**158**
Halibut And Quinoa Mix	**159**
Orange-spiced Pumpkin Hummus	**161**
Artichoke Skewers	**162**
Honey Balsamic Salmon	**163**

Vagus Nerve Practical Guide

Who is the Author

Loren Allen is dedicated to helping others become their best self and live a happy and healthy life. She loves to write and focuses on topics that can make a real difference in helping others accomplish their goals and dreams. She has made it a habit to continue learning new things so that she can share these insights with the world in a concise and helpful way. Loren was born in 1973 and has earned degrees in Business and English with a minor in Psychology.

She has been very successful in the business world for twenty years and is now moving on to her true passion of being a full-time author.Loren has spent much of her life discovering and implementing self-development strategies. Over time, she has become an expert at the best techniques that can really make a difference for a happier and more fulfilling life.

Her favorite role models are Sheryl Sandburg and Oprah Winfrey. Favorite quotes: "Being confident and believing in your own self-worth is necessary to achieving your potential" - Sheryl Sandburg."My philosophy is that not only are you responsible for your life, but doing the best at this moment puts you in the best place for the next moment." - Oprah Winfrey.Loren loves the outdoors and likes to walk or run every day.

She is dedicated to the practice of yoga and feels that meditation is important to both success and happiness. Her driving passion is to pass on to others the knowledge she has gained to make their lives better.

Vagus Nerve Practical Guide

What is Vagus Nerve?

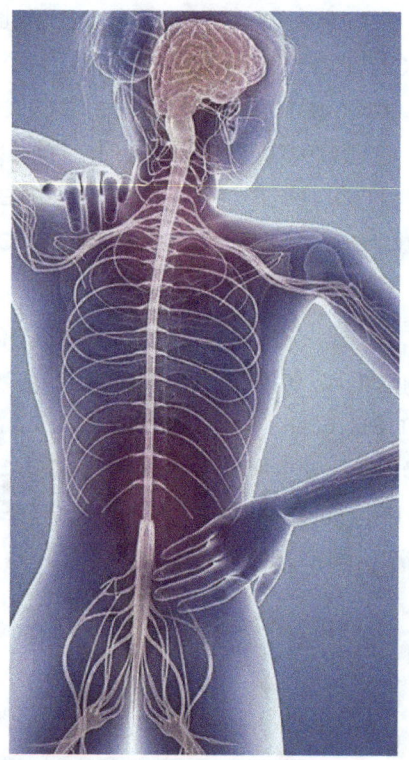

The vagus nerve is responsible for connecting the brain to nearly all of the body's major organs. It runs from the brain stem down each side of the neck, across the chest, and into the abdomen. Additionally, it is linked directly to two regions in consciousness and alertness in different parts of awareness within the brain.

Several researchers have discovered that the vagus nerve can control blood sugar levels without depending on insulin. In fact, this system works for people who don't have diabetes too.

The vagus nerve is a cranial nerve that runs from the brain to the abdomen. It's responsible for sending signals to our nervous system to turn on our bodies' relaxation response, or parasympathetic nervous system.

The vagus nerve is responsible for the release of acetylcholine; a neurotransmitter important for learning and memory.

Acetylcholine not only soothes and relaxes the body, but it also can be used by the vagus nerve to send messages of relaxation and peace throughout your system. In fact, recent studies have found that acetylcholine is a major brake on inflammation in the body.

The vagus nerve is a large, bundle of sensory nerve cell bodies that connects the brainstem to the body. It allows the brain to monitor and receive data on a variety of bodily processes.

The vagus nerve, and its associated structures, provides a variety of nerve system activities. The vagus nerve works in tandem with the sympathetic nervous system to form the free nerve system, which includes parasympathetic and considerate components.

The nerve is responsible for coordinating movement within the body by sending information to and from the brain. It forms a circuit between the neck, lungs, heart, and abdomen.

There are twelve cranial nerves scattered throughout the body. They come in pairs and serve as a link between the brain and other parts of the anatomy, such as the head, neck, and torso. These nerves provide sensory information to the brain relating to smell, sight, taste, and sound.

The cranial nerves that affect sensation are called "sensory." The ones responsible for muscles movement and stimulating different glands are said to have "motor functions."

Some cranial nerves are responsible for sensory or motor functions while others have a combination of both. An example of this is the vagus nerve, which can also be referred to as cranial nerve X. The cranial nerves are grouped and named using Roman numerals depending on what area they're located in.

Anatomical Course

The vagus nerve, which extends from the head to the abdomen, has the longest course of any of the cranial nerves. Its name is derived from the Latin vagari meaning "to wander." It's also known as the "wandering nerve."

In the Mind

The vagus nerve originates from the medulla of the brainstem. It leaves the skull through the jugular foramen along with the glossopharyngeal and accessory nerves.

The auricular branch arises from the skull and supplies sensation to the posterior portion of the external auditory canal and external ear.

In the neck

The vagus nerve enters the carotid sheath at the neck, traveling inferiorly with the internal jugular vein and common carotid artery. The right and left nerves have different pathways at the bottom of the neck:

The left vagus nerve goes into the thorax via a route posterior to the sternoclavicular joint and anterior to the subclavian artery. It passes inferiorly between the left common carotid and left subclavian arteries, posterior to the sternoclavicular joint, going into the thorax on the left side.

Several branches come up from the neck:

The majority of the soft palate muscles and pharynx are innervated by pharyngeal branches.

The superior laryngeal nerve branches off into the external and internal larynx. The cricothyroid muscle, which is responsible for dilating the vocal cords, is innervated by the external larynx. The internal branch provides sensory input to most of the structures in the larynx, including the epiglottis and glottis.

The recurrent laryngeal nerve hooks underneath the right subclavian artery as it rises toward the larynx. It activates most of the intrinsic muscles of the larynx.

In the thorax

The posterior vagal trunk is formed by the right vagus nerve, which runs through the thorax. The anterior vagal trunk is constructed by the left vagus nerve. The oesophageal plexus, which receives nerve fibers from branches of the vagal trunks, helps to develop the smooth muscular tube of the esophagus.

Two different branches come up in the thorax:

The left recurrent laryngeal nerve ascends to innervate most of the intrinsic muscles in the larynx after hooking under the aorta arch.

The role of cardiac branches is to maintain heart rate and send signals for visceral sensation to the organ. The vagal trunks enter through the oesophageal hiatus into the abdomen before opening the diaphragm.

In the abdomen

The vagal trunks in the abdomen divide into branches that supply the esophagus, stomach, and large and small intestines.

Structure and function

The vagus nerve begins in the medulla oblongata and leaves the skull through the jugular foramen, as you can see in Figure 2. It has two ganglia, which are located on the vagus nerve just distal to the inferior ganglion. The spinal accessory nerve connects to the vagus nerve just proximal to the inferior ganglion, whereas it separates from it at approximately one-third of its length.

The nucleus ambiguous, the superior ganglion of X, and the inferior ganglion are responsible for the formation of cell bodies for the vagus nerve. Efferent special visceral fibers originating in the nucleus ambiguous aid in phonation and swallowing modulation.

The fibers within X's dorsal motor nucleus are efferent, general visceral fibers that control organs they innervate and stimulate glands throughout the digestive tract.

The superior ganglion of the vagus nerve provides general somatic innervation to the external ear and tympanic membrane. The inferior ganglion of X provides basic visceral fibers to the aortic bodies and carotid, as well as afferent basic visceral fibers to the aortic bodies and carotid.

The glossopharyngeal nerve is a sensory nerve that conveys taste sensations from the tongue to the pharynx and then to the nucleus tractus solitarius.

The vagus nerve starts its journey by going downward within the carotid sheath. It is located posterior and lateral to the internal and common carotid arteries, and medial to the internal jugular vein.

The vagus nerve branches off into two; the right and left nerves. The right nerve travels in front of the subclavian artery, and then behind the innominate artery before it falls into the thoracic cavity on the right side. It moves past the trachea and hilum until it meets with its partner, forming the esophageal plexus.

The left vagus nerve runs in front of the subclavian artery and enters the thoracic cavity. It then goes down behind the phrenic nerve and posteriorly to the left lung before moving medially towards the esophagus, where it joins with right vagus nerve to form the esophageal plexus.

The vagus nerve has four branches in the neck: pharyngeal, superior laryngeal, recurrent laryngeal, and the superior cardiac nerves.

The pharyngeal nerve emerges from the inferior ganglion of the vagus nerve. This branch contains motor and sensory fibers.

The pharyngeal plexus is formed from these fibers, which shape the pharyngeal plexus, branches of which activate the pharyngeal and palatal muscles, and the pharyngeal plexus also provides innervation to the intercarotid plexus, which receives information from the carotid body.

The superior laryngeal nerve travels between the internal and external carotid arteries and divides into external and internal branches near the hyoid bone. The inner laryngeal nerve passes through the thyrohyoid membrane before entering the larynx.

The external branch of the superior laryngeal nerve accompanies the superior thyroid artery distally. The external branch innervates the cricothyroid muscle, whereas the internal branch supplies mucous membranes more effectively than it does glottis.

The laryngeal nerve fibers on the right side branch from the vagus nerve near the right subclavian artery. They travel upwards to the larynx, passing between the cricopharyngeus muscle and esophagus. The left laryngeal nerve encircles around the aortic arch below where the ligamentum arteriosus is located before entering into thelarynx anatomical structure.

Except for the cricothyroid muscle, all laryngeal muscles are supplied by the recurrent laryngeal nerve. The amazing cardiac nerve, which is connected to parasympathetic fibers and travels to the heart, is released from the vagus nerve while it's within the carotid sheath.

The vagus nerve emits posterior and anterior bronchial branches. The anterior branches are along the anterior lung, forming the anterior pulmonary plexus. The posterior branches form the posterior lung plexus.

The esophageal branches of the vagus nerve form the esophageal plexus. The left vagus is anterior to the esophagus; the right is posterior.

Stomach branches supply the stomach; celiac branches supply the pancreas, adrenals, kidneys, spleen, and small intestine.

What does the vagus nerve affect?

The vagus nerve has various functions, but it is mainly responsible for sensory input from the throat, lungs, heart, and abdomen. It also provides a special taste sensation behind the tongue.

The neck muscles that control swallowing and talking are controlled by the Motor. Its capabilities can be divided into many categories. One of them is to maintain the nervous system in balance.

The nervous system can be thought of as two different sides: the sympathetic and the parasympathetic. The sympathetic side is responsible for increases in alertness, breathing, blood pressure, heart rate, and energy.

The vagus nerve is responsible for the parasympathetic part of the nervous system, which decreases alertness, blood pressure and heart rate. It also promotes relaxation, digestion and calmness. Additionally, the vagus nerve aids with sexual arousal, urination and defecation.

Other vagus nerve effects include:

There is a direct connection between the gut and the brain via the vagus nerve. This nerve delivers information from the gut to the human brain.

The vagus nerve connects to the diaphragm through relaxation techniques. A person gets quite calm when they take deep breaths. The vagus nerve sends an anti-inflammatory alert to other parts of the body.

The vagus nerve is responsible for the heart rate and blood pressure. When it's overactive, it can lead to organ damage and loss of consciousness.

Fear management: the vagus nerve transmits information from the stomach to the brain regarding stress, anxiety, and fear; hence the expression "gut feeling." These messages assist someone in recovering from frightening or stressful events.

Functions of the Vagus Nerve

The vagus nerve has one of the widest distributions of all cranial nerves, with two nerves extending from the brain stem down each side of the body, through the abdominal region, and into the major organs.

The vagus nerve is very complicated, and it helps with many different things like breathing, digestion, and making sure the heartbeat stays regular.

The vagus nerve is responsible for transmitting messages to and from the brain. This includes sensory information from the ears, throat, tongue, windpipe, and voice box.

Disorders that affect the vagus nerve are usually referred to as 10th cranial nerve disorders.

There are several different impacts of these disorders, which can be as complicated as the nerve itself. Some effects are more common than others, for instance if the vagus nerve is stimulated or compressed, it usually results in unconsciousness, crisp skin, and/or nausea.

The vagus nerve can relax the heart and lower blood pressure when stimulated. Although this may appear to be harmful in many instances, the vagus nerve is often stimulated to treat people with severe depression and epilepsy.

The primary function of the vagus nerve is to provide communication between the brain and each of the main organs in the head, neck, chest and abdomen. The gag reflex, heart rate regulation, sweating control, blood pressure management and stimulation of peristalsis are all controlled by this one nerve.

The vagus nerve is a branch of the ninth cranial nerve, which controls the parasympathetic nervous system. Vagus nerves are classified as sensory, motor, specialized sensory, and parasympathetic fibers. Although it is mostly an afferent nerve that conveys sensations from the body to the brain, the vagus nerve is also an efferent nerve that transmits information from the brain to muscles.

The parasympathetic nervous system controls smooth muscle control.

Four separate vagal passageways exit from the medulla oblongata:

Dorsal nucleus: sends parasympathetic information to the viscera

The tongue furnishes sensory information to a single nucleus. The back trigeminal nucleus, also known as the trigeminal nerve, is a part of the spine that receives sensory input from the outer ear and laryngeal mucosa.

The motor nerve that controls swallowing, talking, and heart muscle activity is a potential nucleus. The gray matter of cranial nerve nuclei represents the synaptic strain.

The vagus nerve relays messages to and from the brain through synapses in the medulla oblongata. Other nerves in the body follow a similar pattern, with messages being sent back and forth between different parts of the body before reaching their final destination.

The vagus nerve provides sensation to the skin and mucous membranes of the external ear, throat, and voice box. It also allows an individual to feel pain, vibration, distension, and nausea in visceral organs.

For example, the autonomic nervous system sends involuntary signals in reaction to specific chemical stimuli such as hormones and neurotransmitters. The visceral organs include heart, pancreas, liver lungs and intestines.

The vagus nerve, as the only sensory nerve on the epiglottis and tongue, collects data from those feeling buds. CN X is a motor nerve that activates the throat's muscles. After a serious struggle, the parasympathetic nervous system has a spontaneous resting function that helps to bring the body to a more peaceful state. There is no need for flight reaction for survival.

The vagus nerve, which is a component of the parasympathetic nervous system, innervates the heart's smooth muscles, the trachea, the bronchi of the lungs, and the gastrointestinal tract. It will slow down heart rate and breathing if encouraged.

The Vasovagal Reflex

The vagus nerve is responsible for the "vasovagal reflex," which is a sudden drop in blood pressure and heart rate. This can be caused by an intestinal illness, reaction to pain, or fright/stress.

People who are especially susceptible to vasovagal reflexes may experience a drop in blood pressure and heart rate that can cause them to faint—a condition called "vasovagal syncope."

Vagus nerve activation is commonly associated with dysautonomias.

Stimulating the vagus nerve may help doctors detect particular murmurs by helping to break episodes of supraventricular tachycardia and might assist them in diagnosing specific heart-type murmurs. Vagal stimulation is simple to achieve with the Valsalva maneuver.

The Vagus Nerve and the Heart

The vagus nerve is responsible for supplying the sinus node and when stimulated, it can produce sinus bradycardia. The left vagus nerve supplies the AV node and its stimulation can create a heart block. By producing a transient heart block, the Valsalva maneuver can be terminated.

The Role of Vagus in the Autonomic Nervous System

The parasympathetic nervous system, which includes the sympathetic and inhibitory nerves, is made up of three branches: the voluntary (sympathetic) and involuntary (inhibitory) nerves.

The anatomical significance of the sympathetic and parasympathetic nervous systems is what most people are familiar with. The vagus nerve will be the major source of the parasympathetic nervous system. The nervus oculomotorius, nervus glossopharyngeus, and nervus facialis are the other parasympathetic cranial nerves.

The vagus nerve is most notable for being afferent, which means it relays information from the internal organs to the brain. This suggests that the gut, heart, liver, and lungs are significant sources of sensory input for the mind.

The intestines are probably the most extended surface toward the exterior world and may be an extremely sensitive sense organ in its own right.

The vagus nerve has been investigated as an eccentric nerve and the arch-enemy of the sympathetic nervous system. The vagus nerve sends parasympathetic divergence to most organs, which are then controlled by efferents from the splanchnics.

The parasympathetic nervous system, which is made up of two branches, controls vegetative functions by counteracting one another. The parasympathetic innervation causes bronchioles and capillaries to dilate and saliva glands to be stimulated.

The innervation of the sympathetic nervous system leads to a constriction of capillaries, dilatation of bronchioles, increased heart rate and tightness in the digestive tract and urinary sphincters. In the intestinal tract, activating the parasympathetic nervous system increases glandular secretion and bowel motility.

On the other hand, understanding calms the digestive system's reduction of blood flow to the gut. This allows more circulation to muscles and the heart when they are under stress.

The Enteric Nervous System (ENS) is a collection of nerve cells that originate from the vagal neural crest cells. These nerves form a plexus within the walls of the gastrointestinal tract, running the entire length of it from the esophagus to anal canal. Scientists believe that there are approximately 100-500 million neurons in an ENS.

The Enteric Nervous System (ENS) is a collection of nerve cells in the body that plays a similar role to the brain in terms of chemical coding, function, and structure. Because of this, it has been nicknamed the "second brain" or the "mind within the gut."

The abdominal wall contains two ganglionated plexuses, one in the submucosal layer and one in the myenteric plexus (or innermost layer) that controls gastrointestinal blood flow, regulates epithelial cell secretion and function, and manages digestive wall relaxation and contraction.

The ENS is responsible for digestive tract procedures, like microvascular flow and epithelial secretion of fluid, ions, and bioactive peptides. It also plays a role in immune system function and nutrient absorption.

The ENS is directly linked to the vagal nerve, and the crucial transmitter is cholinergic activation via nicotinic receptors. The connection between the ENS and the vagal nerve as components of the brain causes a two-way flow of information.

On the other hand, ENS can function independently of vagal control even in the large and small intestines. It comprises functional reflex pathways, including sensory, motor, and nerve cells. They are in charge of muscle activity and motility as well as mucosal blood flow and barrier functionality.

As a result, the ENS will continue to maintain close contact with both innate and adaptive immune system cells, monitoring their activities and services. The Cell Lobe ENS is concerned with issues such as incontinence and constipation.

If the ENS fails in either the large or small intestine, it could be life-threatening, whereas losing the vagal nerve would not have such severe consequences.

The vagus nerve is a link between the central and ENS. The bidirectional connection between the mind and gastrointestinal tract is made possible by the connection between the ENS and the CNS.

It's in charge of maintaining physiological homeostasis and linking the brain's cognitive and emotional areas with peripheral intestinal activities such as immune activation, enteric reflex, intestinal permeability, and enteroendocrine communication.

The brain-gut axis is made up of the brain, the spinal cord, the free nervous system, and the hypothalamic-pituitary-adrenal (HPA) axis. Vagus efferents send signals from beneath the brain to the gut through efferent fibers, which make up 10–20% of all threads, and vagus afferents from the digestive wall to the brain account for 80–90 percent of all fibers.

The autonomic nervous system's vagal efferent pathways are related to the HPA axis, which controls an organism's changes in response to any type of stress. Specifically, environmental stress and high circulating pro-inflammatory cytokines stimulate the secretion of corticotropin-releasing factor from the hypothalamus, thus turning on the HPA axis.

The CRF stops the release of adrenocorticotropic hormone from the pituitary gland. Cortisol is a potent stress hormone that affects multiple human organs, including the brain, muscles, bones, and body fat.

The brain is able to control the function of intestinal cells like immune cells, epithelial cells, enteric neurons, smooth muscle interstitial cells of Cajal enterochromaffin cells through both hormonal and neural communication.

The gut microbiota has the opposite effect on these cells, impacting the brain-gut axis by communicating with intestinal cells and ENS. This influence directly impacts metabolic systems and neuroendocrine function.

The microbiota has been linked to mood, anxiety, and depressive-like symptoms in previous research. The microbiota has been discovered to affect stress reactivity and anxiety-like behavior as well as the set point for HPA activity in germ-free animals in studies.

Consequently, these animals commonly show decreased anxiety and increased stress responses with augmented cortisol and ACTH levels.

The vagus nerve, which runs from the brain to the stomach, plays a role in regulating digestion. Vagal afferents send info about food intake and calorie consumption to the brain, helping to determine how quickly nutrients are absorbed and stored.

Visceral afferent endings of the Vagus Nerve in the intestinal tract express a wide range of chemical and mechanosensitive receptors, as shown by electrophysiological and histological evidence.

In response to nutrients through distension of the stomach and neuronal signals, enteroendocrine cells of the intestinal system release regulatory peptides and gut hormonal chemicals such as trophic factors. These receptors are targets of inhibitory neurotransmitters and neuropeptide Y released from enteroendocrine cells in the digestive tract in response to meals.

The hormones mentioned below affect an individual's food intake by communicating with thepart of the brain responsible for satiety, gastric emptying, and energy balance.

The nutrient content of the stomach is also dangerous to many hormones, including peptide cholecystokinin. They are involved in short-term emotions of gratification and hunger regulation. Cholecystokinin activates CCK 1 receptors on vagal afferent fibers innervating the gut, which controls gastrointestinal activities such as stomach emptying and food intake by activating them.

Furthermore, CCK is key for secreting pancreatic fluid and producing gastric acid. It also aids in gallbladder contraction, decreased gastric emptying, and digestion facilitation. Saturated fat, long-chain fats from amino acids and small peptides derived from protein play a part in exciting CCK's release from the bowels.

The biologically active forms of CCK, which are classified by the number of amino acids they contain, include CCK-22, CCK-8, and CCK-5. i.e., and 33 are examples of these biologically active forms.

In contrast, the endocrine gut cells contain a combination of more significant and small CCK peptides, with CCK 22 or CCK 33 often dominating. In rats, long and short-chain fatty acids from food activate jejunal vagal afferent nerve fibers through separate mechanisms.

Short-chain fats, such as butyric acid, have an immediate effect on vagal afferent terminals. Meanwhile, long-chain fatty acids activatevagal afferents through a CCK-dependent system.

By exogenously administering CCK, it seems to prevent the body's natural production of CCK.CCK is a neurotransmitter found in enteric vagal afferent neurons in various areas of the brain, including the cerebral cortex, thalamus, hypothalamus, basal ganglia and dorsal hindbrain. When CCK activates vagal afferent terminals in the NTS , this results in an increase of calcium release.

Finally, there's evidence that CCK can activate neurons in the hindbrain and myenteric intestinal plexus in rats. That capsaicin or vagotomy therapy reduces CCK-induced Fos expression in the brain. There's also plenty of proof that high levels of CCK induce anxiety.

Consequently, it is difficult to model stress and anxiety disorders in animals and people using CCK.

Ghrelin is another hormone that Is released into the bloodstream from the stomach. It stimulates appetite by preventing a vagal nerve impulses. Ghrelin levels are increased when an individual is fasting and decrease after eating a meal.

Acylated ghrelin, when administered peripherally or centrally, stimulates food intake and growth hormone secretion in rats. Chronic administration leads to weight gain.

In rats that have been treated or vagotomized with capsaicin, a specific afferent neurotoxin, the feeding action of ghrelin is diminished or perhaps shut down. In humans, subcutaneous injection or intravenous infusion result in increased hunger and food desires as ghrelin inhibits insulin production.

As a result, it's not surprising that secretion is disrupted in obesity and insulin resistance. Leptin receptors have also been found in the vagus nerve. In rodents, leptin and CCK appear to work together to promote short-term inhibition of long-term food consumption and weight loss.

The epithelial cells that respond to both ghrelin and leptin are located near the vagal mucosal endings, and they modulate the activity of vagal afferents. In other words, these cells work together to regulate food consumption. However, after diet-induced obesity and fasting in mice, leptin is no longer able to effectively influence vagal mucosal afferents.

The gastrointestinal tract may sense basic tastes similarly to how the tongue does, by way of G-protein-coupled taste receptors. The release of various gastric peptides occurs when different tastes are present.

The release of CCK can be used to minimize appetite by targeting bitter taste receptors. Furthermore, the activation of bitter taste receptors promotes ghrelin production and so affects the vagus nerve.

What Happens If The Vagus Nerve Is Damaged?

It is also conceivable that the vagus nerve can be damaged. It's possible that excessive pressure or stress on the nerve might cause it to be destroyed. If stimulation isn't done correctly, it may induce damage if done repetitively.

A break in a nerve can be caused by surgical instruments as well, and it's not uncommon for surgeons to accidentally damage or cut nerves during surgery. Regardless, damage to nerves may have serious consequences for the patient.

If your nerve is completely damaged, you may experience some of the following problems.

· Speaking or Voice Problems: When nerves are damaged, it can cause hoarseness or make it difficult to speak.

· Trouble Eating and Drinking: Any damage to the vagus nerve may disrupt how your throat muscles operate. This will, eventually, give you trouble with taking food or swallowing water.

In other words, vagus nerve damage mainly impacts your gag reflex. As we have seen, the gag reflex is responsible for making sure that your food pipe stays open so you can swallow food as you eat.

· Loss of Hearing or Pain in the Ear: The vagus nerve is responsible for communicating messages between the brain and various organs in the body, so damage to this nerve can result in pain or hearing loss.

The nerve is also connected to your eardrums directly. This implies that any damage to the nerve might have an effect on your hearing and result in deafness or ear discomfort.

· Affected Heart Rate and Blood Pressure: The vagus nerve is the extension of the autonomic nervous system that directly links the heart to the brain. When this vital connection is damaged, your heart rate and blood pressure will be greatly affected.

Vagus nerve stimulation has been shown to promote the development of brain circuitry and improve heart-brain coordination. VNS does this by altering communication between neurons in the brain and those in the heart. It can have a strong influence on how well your heart beats and how fast it does so.

The heart rate and blood pressure are interconnected--a faster heartbeat will result in higher blood pressure, while a steadier heartbeat leads to lower blood pressure.

· Abdominal Pains and Stomach Pains: The vagus nerve is susceptible to injury. The result of this is that stomach acids may be decreased. This implies that you might have trouble digesting food. At all times, a minimum level of stomach acid should be maintained in the stomach.

Damage to the vagus nerve means that there is no signal from the stomach glands indicating that they should begin acid production. In addition, any damage to the vagus nerve may also impact abdominal muscles.

The vagus nerve, in collaboration with the nervous system, innervates the abdominal area. The nerve is responsible for sexual arousal because it extends to all the sexual parts. The nerve sends signals that start ovulation and other sexual activities.

When damage occurs to the nerve, there is a higher likelihood that abdominal pain will be experienced, especially by women.

Communication Effects of Vagus Nerve Damage

The auricular vagus nerve is the connection from the brain's central vagus nerve to the ear. It terminates on the back of the ear, where it branches off into smaller nerves that innervate different parts of the ear.

This nerve is responsible for collecting communication senses and sending signals to the brain for interpretation. In other words, it plays an important role in processing sensory information.

If the vagus nerve was not placed appropriately, this would be a major problem for the majority of people. If the vagus nerve is damaged, you may experience one or more of the following symptoms:

Inability to Perceive Words:

We not only glean information from what we hear audibly, but also through observation. For example, you can often tell what a person is saying by watching their lips move. In many ways, these additional observations help to connect the voice of the speaker with the words they are saying, making communication more straightforward and seamless.

If the vagus nerve is entirely damaged, however, then we lose the sensory hearing aspect. In other words, we can't relate the movements of another person's mouth directly to their voice.

When words are not exchanged for communication, it often leads to complications. In these cases, it is vital to have sharp observation skills so that you can interpret what the person is saying without relying on hearing their words.

Inability to Perceive the Direction of Voices:

One way that human beings can maintain a clear focus in life is by being able to sense the direction of a voice. If you're surrounded by voices but don't know which way they're coming from, it can be very confusing and difficult to manage.

A balance of voices is necessary to help a person stay upright and stable. If there are any imbalances in hearing, it may cause leaning or tilting. For example, damage to the vagus nerves in one ear can force a person to tilt towards the side where that sense is still active.

The ability to hear the direction of a voice is important in many aspects of communication. For example, if your ears are unable to detect the direction from which a sound is coming while you're conversing with many individuals at once, you won't be able to perform effectively.

If you work at a speed where conversation flows down a chain, you might have difficulties linking up the chain. When traveling across streets, the most hazardous situation for a person suffering from vagus nerve damage is hearing in which direction the sound is coming from.

Road accidents can easily happen if you cannot determine the location of a sound. It may take longer to identify an oncoming car, or you might run into danger thinking it is coming from the other direction.

The vagus nerve is integral to communication, meaning it's essential that the nerve remains healthy. If the nerve fails, it can result in many issues at a personal level.

Inability to Perceive High Volumes:

Individuals with a damaged vagus nerve might not be able to detect the volume of sounds, though they can still hear them.

Because of the very long duration it takes for epinephrine to be absorbed into the bloodstream, patients who are not allergic to anti-inflammatory agents may inadvertently receive extremely high doses without realizing. This is a significant risk since it can result in eardrum damage as a result of the large amounts. The vagus nerve is essential for keeping the ears safe from loud noises and high volumes. Without healthy sensory nerves, it's impossible to tell the difference between sounds.

Without the proper stimuli, the ear cannot warn the brain of potential dangers. This leaves patients susceptible to accidents that could damage their eardrums and cause a total loss of hearing.

You also lose a lot of information if you can't see quantities. You must notice actions and tone when interacting with someone. If a person's voice rises during an argument or discussion, you may hear that they're becoming emotional based on the changed pitch.

Your vagus nerve is essential for detecting communication flaws; without a nerves to detect them, you wouldn't be able to understand voice variations. This is why it's important to protect your vagus nerve from any damage.

Pain in the Ear:

In addition to disruptions in communication, another tell-tale sign that your vagus nerve is damaged is continuous pain in the ear. While this doesn't necessarily affect hearing, if left untreated the pain could result in other serious problems. If you've been experiencing an aching sensation in your ear or along the veins leading to it, it's likely due to damage of the vagus nerve.

When the auricular nerves are damaged, people frequently report suffering from ear discomfort that extends to the neck. The auricular nerve connects your neck and head together; any damage to your ear nerves may also affect your neck and head.

If the vagus nerve in your ear is damaged, it can lead to pain in your neck and headaches. This can affect your concentration and cause hearing problems over time. You may feel like there is something blocking your ears.

When you're in pain, it's tough to hold a conversation. Most people who have damaged nerves stay in discomfort for an extended period of time. When they try to speak, they often wonder if the other person is actually understanding them.

The Response of the Body When the Nerve is Damaged

The vagus nerve is a major actor in our internal and external bodies. Should the vagus nerve be damaged, several essential body areas will lose their sense. We know that the vagus nerve gives two types of sensory reaction through its action on the brainstem.

The somatic component of the vagus nerve refers to the external sensory sensation provided by the nerve. The external senses of the vagus nerve are mainly felt on the skin or in muscles. In areas where the vagus nerve extends to the surface of your skin, you may be able to feel a sensation associated with it. A good example is an ear, where auricular nerves extend to its surface.

The vagus nerve is responsible for providing the viscera (internal organs) with information. The term "visceral sense" refers to a third sensory function carried out by the vagus nerve. This is mostly concerned with internal bodily organs' perceptions. In essence, the vagus nerve has control over some of our most essential internal body organs, and it is accountable for their reaction time when they are called upon to respond quickly.

A vagus nerve that isn't functioning correctly can interfere with both the somatic and visceral systems in a person's body. This nerve plays an important role in not only keeping people alert, but also helping their internal organs function properly.

The nerve's ability to detect changes in the body and promote the production of essential hormones makes it essential for normal bodily function. If the vagus nerve is damaged, any individual would be unable to live a typical existence due to its sensory capabilities.

Some of the symptoms associated with a damaged vagus nerve are due to sensory loss. In a patient who has had a vagotomy, it is probable that the vagus nerve will not stimulate intestinal glands to release stomach acids when required.

Consequently, a person may have acid reflux, vomiting and nausea to name a few issues. Also, we have found that those with a damaged vagus nerve often lack appetite or vomit not long after eating.

All of this is due to the fact that the glands that produce enzymes and acids do not receive the proper signal from the brain. Any damage to the vagus nerve can have an effect on any of the following bodily organs and regions.

Affected body parts

The Ear:

Hearing loss can be caused by a variety of things, including age-related hearing loss (presbycusis), ear infections, and damage to the inner ear. The auricular vagus nerve, which extends all the way to the outside of the ear's outer skin, might be damaged. This is because if a person has an injured nerve, their ears may not be able to feel any sensation or hear sounds at times.

The vagus nerve, which originates in the ear and runs to the ear canal, acts as a connection between the brain and various organs. Even without a person detecting pain, damage to the ear canal may occur as a result of this relationship. Communication is also influenced by all of these elements, as demonstrated above.

To keep your hearing ability, you must safeguard your vagus nerve from harm. We have already examined some of the causes of ear canal damage.

The points below will help you keep your ears safe from damage. We will also explore some natural ways to protect your vagus nerve as we go along.

Throat:

Another location in the body that may be affected by a vagus nerve disorder is the respiratory system. The vagus nerve runs from the ear to the throat. It's the vagus nerve that enables gag reflex, which is a vital bodily function.

It's difficult for anyone to chew and swallow food when a gag reflex is absent. The damage to your vagus nerve might cause throat muscles to fail, resulting in chewing and swallowing difficulties.

Visceral Sensation for the Larynx:

The larynx (voice box) is a critical component in your communication. The well-being of the vagus nerve affects this body part's reaction the most. If your vagus nerve is badly damaged, you may not be able to communicate successfully.

In other words, a damaged vagus nerve may directly affect your speech. Some people who have damaged vagus nerves produce wheezy voices while others completely fail to speak. The greater the damage to the nerve, the less ability that person has to communicate verbally. If the damage is severe, a person may be completely inaudible when they speak.

Sensory Effect for the Esophagus:

The esophageal (eh-so-fuh-jee-uhl) nerve is a extension of the vagus nerve that goes to the esophagus. This nerve is very important in sending communications to the brain and back to the esophagus. The vagus nerve plays an important role in directing food down to the stomach.

If the esophagus does not have a sensory impact, then food ingested will not descend to the stomach. To assist in the movement of food as it is lowered into the stomach, the esophagus is always being squeezed.

All of these movements are subliminally directed by the vagus nerve. If there is damage to the vagus nerve, it would cause trouble since a person would have to put forth great effort to push food into their stomach.

Sensory Action in the Lungs:

The lungs play a crucial role in your body, and any damage to the vagus nerve can have an effect on them. Not only do they help you breathe, but they also circulate fresh air to the brain.

The unconscious movement of air into and out of the lungs is controlled by the vagus nerve. This nerve regulates the rate of blood vessel contraction and expansion. If this function is disrupted, it could result in difficultly breathing and a host of other problems.

Sensory Action in the Trachea:

The trachea, commonly known as the windpipe, is a vital bodily structure that connects your throat to your lungs. We've said that the gag reflex in your throat causes food and air to be separated at the throat. You've undoubtedly been in a situation where tiny remnants of food have made it into your trachea.

If you inhale even a very small piece of food, it can cause extensive coughing and suffocation. If action is not taken within a few minutes, the person may choke to death. This highlights how delicate the trachea is. The vagus nerve sensory action helps distinguish between the esophagus and trachea.

The vagus nerve directs food to the esophagus while controlling air movement in and out of the trachea.

All of these factors would be affected in the event of a vagus nerve injury. The trachea would fail to synchronize breathing activities, resulting in issues.

Sensory Action to the Heart:

The heart is a vital organ, and the thought of damage to the vagus nerve (which directly coordinates its actions) is chilling.

The pulmonary and cardiac extensions of the vagus nerve directly coordinate the activities of the heart. The activities of the heart are controlled subconsciously by the vagus nerve, meaning that the vagus nerve can coordinate the actions of the heart without your input.

The cardiac activity, blood vessel constriction, and communication between the heart and brain are all activities of the vagus nerve that may be detected by touch. These activities can have a quick influence on the heart rate and blood pressure, as we have already seen. Any damage to the vagus nerve might disrupt the regular operations of the heart.

Regular activities may be curtailed or may take an abnormal course. Overstimulation of the vagus nerve has been shown to result in a decrease in blood pressure and an increase in heart rate. A damaged nerve, therefore, might also cause a considerable reduction in heart pressure.

The following actions may lead to fainting. If the condition worsens, the vagus nerve might become irreparably damaged. As a result, the person might slip into a permanent state of unconsciousness.

The Functions of the Nervous System

Sensation

We take in our surroundings through our senses--touch, sight, sound, smell or taste. After we interact with something from the outside world, it's our nervous system's job to get that information and help us understand what's going on around us.

While our sense of touch and sound help us to understand physical stimuli, taste and smell aid in the detection of chemical stimuli. Our sight is triggered by light.

What would happen if you were crossing railroad tracks and couldn't hear the approaching train? What would it be like if you couldn't tell whether your bath water was too cold or hot?

Our senses give us the capacity to interact safely with our surroundings by detecting potential harmful stimuli and allowing us to avoid them. Our brain can't accurately interpret or recognize what we're exposed to if our sensory organs aren't working properly. The sensation of stimuli is one of the most essential features of the nervous system since it allows other functions to function.

Response

The body's natural response to stimuli is illustrated in this simple example. Sweating is produced as a natural cooling mechanism when the body senses an increase in temperature; this is why you are more likely to sweat on a hot day than a cold one.

Danny sees a butterfly. The stimulus is then perceived and identified in his brain before he responds to it.

When we interact with the outside world, a signal is sent to the brain so that we may identify what we are seeing, after which comes the reaction, which is determined by the stimulus detected.

In Danny's situation, the butterfly attracts him, so he rushes after it; but when he sees the local dog, his instinct tells him to flee since he has identified a potential hazard.

The nervous system allows the body to sense, process and respond to stimuli in a cyclical pattern. Neurons transmit signals from the body's sensory organs to the brain, where the information is processed. The brain then sends signals back to the glands and muscles, telling them how to respond.

Conscious responses, or voluntary responses, are controlled by the somatic nervous system and occur when we contract our skeletal muscles. For example, Danny running after the butterfly is a voluntary response.

Involuntary responses differ from voluntary ones in that they're characterized by the activation of glands and muscles which we don't have conscious control over. The autonomic nervous system is responsible for governing these involuntary processes-- sweating being one example.

Integration

The nervous system is in charge of getting information from the environment through our senses, which we need to process and understand before reacting. This reactive function is known as integration.

By constantly compare what we see and experience with our previous memories, we form our perception of the world around us. This understanding then directs how we respond to certain stimuli.

The Cranial Nerves

The cranial and spinal nerves form the peripheral nerve system, which connects various bodily organs via the brain and spine. The brain gives rise to the cranial nerves, which exit the skull at its base. Cranial nerves include sensory and motor neurons, but some are solely sensory.

There are cranial nerves all with different functions. These nerves are:

· The Olfactory nerve which controls our sense of smell

· The Optic nerve which regulates vision

· The Oculomotor (okuhl-oh-motor) nerve which regulates the movement of the eyeballs and eyelids.

· The Trochlear (troh-klee-uh) nerve which regulates eye movement

· The Trigeminal nerve which controls chewing and facial sensations.

· The Abducens (ab-dew-sens) nerve which controls eye movement.

· The Facial nerve which controls our facial expressions as well as our sense of taste.

· The Vestibulocochlear (veh-sti-bew-low-koch-lee-uh) nerve which regulates balance and hearing.

· The Glossopharyngeal nerve is responsible for three functions: controlling the secretion of saliva, sense of taste and swallowing.

· The Vagus nerve which regulates even muscles and motor responses in the heart lungs and throat.

· The Accessory nerve which regulates neck and shoulder movement.

· The Hypoglossal nerve, which controls both speech and tongue movement as well as swallowing.

The vestibulocochlear nerve, optic nerve, and olfactory nerve are all sensory nerves. They control our eyesight, smell, and hearing abilities. A difficulty with nerve VIII, for example, would indicate a problem with the vestibulocochlear nerve; which controls both our hearing and balance.

The optic nerve is responsible for our peripheral and central vision while the olfactory nerve manages our sense of smell. To test if the olfactory nerve is working properly, close one nostril and inhale different scents with the other.

The motor nerves control numerous bodily functions. The oculomotor, trochlear, abducens, hypoglossal, and accessory nerves are all examples of motor nerves. The hypoglossal nerve regulates speech and tongue movement natural for a person.

The accessory nerve controls shoulder and neck movement, while the oculomotor, trochlear and abducens nerves regulate eye movement.

There are sensory and motor nerves in the brain, which are referred to as mixed nerves. Vagus, trigeminal, glossopharyngeal, and facial are all mixed nerves with both sensory and motor capabilities.

The trigeminal nerve is the cranial nerve responsible for facial sensation, corneal responses, and chewing. It is made of ophthalmic (of-thal-muhk), mandibular, and maxillary nerves.

The facial nerve is responsible for movement in the face, as well as taste and sense of smell. The symmetry of the face or its lack can be used to evaluate the facial nerve. The glossopharyngeal nerve controls saliva flow, taste perception, and swallowing mechanics.

The Vagus nerve is responsible for regulating motor control of the digestive system, as well as regulated muscle sensory in the heart, lungs, and throat.

How to know if your Vagus nerve is injured or compressed

Damage to your nerves might influence the capacity of your brain to communicate with your muscles and organs. Fringe neuropathy is inflammation of the fringe nerves. Damage can be caused by stretching or pushing on a nerve. The nerves may also be damaged as a result of other health conditions that affect the nerves, such as diabetes or Guillain-Barre (gee-yan-bah-re) syndrome.

Carpal tunnel syndrome is caused by pressure on the median nerve in the wrist. This pressure can be from obesity or, occasionally, from an injury such as playing sports or being in a car accident. In some cases of peripheral nerve damage, either the nerves themselves or the protective sheath around them are damaged but these wounds usually heal over time.

In increasingly severe peripheral nerve wounds, both the filaments and protection are damaged, resulting in a complete cut of the nerve. These types of injuries are tough to heal because they are so damaging to the nerves.

Nerve damage can cause several symptoms, the most notable of which are numbness and tingling. You may have harmed at least one nerve during a fall if you feel shivering, lifelessness, or have a limb, arm, shoulder, or hand problem. If a nerve is being packed because of factors like a restricted path tumor or other diseases, you might experience comparable side effects.

If you severely damage a nerve, you may completely lose feeling in the area where the nerve is injured. That's why it's crucial to get medical attention for peripheral nerve damage as soon as possible—there's a chance that the tissue can be repaired. Early diagnosis and treatment sometimes can prevent complications and permanent damage.

Signs your vagal nerve is powerless

The vagal nerve can become weak or irritated due to exposure to poisonous metals, poor posture, hiatal hernias, excessive alcohol consumption, stress, and brain injury (a single concussion can cause weakened vagal nerve tone).

The following symptoms can be caused by indications of powerless vagal nerve tone or mismanaged Vagal Nerve Discharge termination:

·Lack of a muffle reflex

·Slow absorption of nourishment sits in your stomach excessively long. This can cause heartburn or GERD, swelling, or clogging.

·Inability to unwind

·Heart palpitations

·Insomnia

Probably the best indication of solid vagal tone is the point at which your pulse increments somewhat with inward breath, and moderates marginally with exhalation.

How would you reinforce the vagal nerve?

The hereditary component of 60% contributes to our expression, whereas 40% is within our control! Learn about several techniques for strengthening and revitalizing the vagus nerve.

You should keep in mind that two milliliters is the usual amount of blood collected at one time. In fact, it takes approximately 2 million times this volume to make enough blood for a single person!

When you are under a lot of stress, your vagus nerve becomes revitalized and your pulse drops rapidly, making you feel dizzy or forgetful. It's only brief, so don't worry if you miss it!

Frightful vagal nerve tone is linked to irritation, dejection, loneliness, and cardiovascular problems. It's critical that our vagal nerves remain healthy! The following all invigorate the vagus nerve sufficiently enough to be very therapeutic without being excessively restorative. Furthermore, these are not particularly distressing events.

1. Gargling

Gargling activates the vagus nerve, but a gentle swishing won't suffice. You must wash noisily and forcefully, to the point of nearly choking. Doing this daily will help improve your vagal nerve's responsiveness to promote relaxation, detoxification, digestion and more.

2. Playing instruments

Playing a didgeridoo was found to be beneficial in treating obstructive rest syndrome and sleep apnea, according on studies conducted with the instrument. More study has shown that various provocative circumstances also improved. The vagus nerve is generally activated by wind instruments.

3. Yogic or Deep Breathing

Animating the vagus nerve is easy--all you have to do is hold your breath for 6-8 counts. Try this: Inhale through your stomach for a count of 6, hold for 6-8, and then exhale gradually through pursed lips over another 6-8 counts.

It's necessary to be able to feel your stomach expanding with every breath. This 10-minute breathing exercise activates the vagal nerve, which has a calming effect.

4. Meditation

Learning to cherish and be grateful for the positive reflections in our lives improves vagal tone. This is because it strengthens our positive feelings and associations. The more positive we feel, the stronger our vagal tone becomes.

Vagus Nerve: How to invigorate it

The vagus nerve is the longest cranial never, and it starts in the brain just behind the ears. This nerve is responsible for managing most of the body's major organs.

The Cerebral Spinal System (CNS) is the network that runs through your body and connects each organ to your brain. It transmits signals from your cerebral stem to almost all of your instinctive organs, and it's essentially the CEO of your internal operational centre, giving nerve driving power to each organ in your body.

The word vagus actually means "wanderer", since it wanders all throughout the body from the brain down to the reproductive organs, hitting everything in between. In terms of mind-body connection, the vagus nerve is incredible, since it reaches all of the major organs except for the adrenal and thyroid glands.

This nerve is responsible for communicating between the brain and all the organs it's in contact with. Additionally, it helps to control emotions such as anxiety and sadness. Our social interactions are closely related to the vagus nerve because it affects the nerves that help us hear speech, make eye contact, and controls movement of our facial muscles needed for expressions like smiling.

It has the power to impact genuine hormone release in the body, which keeps our psychological and physical structures healthy.

The vagus nerve is responsible for increasing stomach causticity and producing stomach juice to assist with the digestion process. It can also aid you in absorbing vitamin B12 when active.

When you're having problems with it, you may develop genuine gut concerns like Colitis, IBS, and Re-transition. In light of the fact that it is controlled by the vagus nerve, re-motion issues are due to a vagus nerve defect. Gerd and re-motion are caused by an inappropriate throat response.

Without the vagus nerve, we would be more prone to diseases such as heart attacks and diabetes. The vagus nerve helps control our pulse and blood pressure, which in turn prevents us from developing coronary illness. It also balances our blood sugar levels in the liver and pancreas, helping to prevent diabetes.

The vagus nerve, which is the longest of all nerve roots, carries bile from the gallbladder to the rest of your body. It's this nerve that advances general kidney function and expands blood flow, allowing our bodies to filter more efficiently.

At this point, the vagus nerve will reach the spleen and irritation in all observable organs will be reduced. This nerve also has the power to regulate fertility and climaxes in ladies. A dormant or blocked vagus nerve can wreak havoc on your entire brain and body.

The vagus nerve is responsible for the proper function of all major organs, so it stands to reason that any mental or physical illness can be cured by stimulating the vagus nerve.

On issues such as anxiety, heart disease, cerebral pains and headaches, fibromyalgia, alcohol addiction, training course problems, gastrointestinal issues, memory concerns, disposition difficulties , MS, and a variety of other serious illnesses.

There are many archived approaches to animate the vagus nerve, for example:

-Singing or reciting

-Giggling

-Yoga

-Contemplation

-Breathing activities

-Training

Singing and giggling work the muscles at the back of your throat which actuates the nerve.

The vagus nerve is normally strengthened by moderate exercise and training as a general rule increases gut liquids, implying that the vagus nerve has been invigorated. A controlled Yoga practice can also enhance the action of this nerve due to the gains, but it also activates the Meditation and OM-ing.

Utilize these trigged animations to stimulate the vagus nerve:

In April of this year, researchers from the University of Toronto, Wilfrid Laurier University, and Baycrest Center Hospital conducted an inquiry into individuals with Alzheimer's Disease. Patients with various phases of Alzheimer's disease were studied by analysts from the University of Toronto, Wilfrid Laurier University, and Baycrest Center Hospital in an attempt to verify sound re-enactment at 40 hertz.

The researchers found "encouraging" results with clarity, awareness, and readiness. Lee Bartel, one of the brains behind these findings stated that,"The recurrence rate in the brain appears to be around 40 Hz, and parts of it give off the feeling of being at a similar recurring incident.

In other words, when you have a lack of sleep, the parts of your brain that need to communicate with one another - like the thalamus and hippocampus - won't be able to. The result is that you won't be able to form long-term memories."

Bartel explained that the sound-recreation treatment at 40 Hz produces an "expanded" recurrence, which allows "portions of the mind to communicate with one another again."

The inventor of the technique, Alfred A Tomatis (o-tow-lahrin-gohlow-jist), was a French otolaryngologist who believed that the ear's most important function is to provide electrical incitement to every one of the cells in the body, "conditioning up" the whole structure and giving greater energy to people. (Tomatis. 1978)

Tomatis argued that high-pitched music is invigorating while lower tones are calming, and he believed that he could treat a variety of illnesses through sound therapy.

The Tomatis Method has been shown to be an effective treatment for a variety of issues, including depression, ADD, ADHD, and OCD.

"When compared with the non-Tomatis control group, the Tomatis group's results showed factually significant improvements in handling speed, phonological mindfulness, phonemic unravelling competence when reading, conduct, and sound-related thinking."

Sound is increasingly becoming one of the most popular natural healing methods today! It is a great tool to use for stimulating the vagus nerve, and promoting the health and vitality of all organs in your body.

Through sound mending and Crystal Chakra Singing Bowls, you may do this. It is thought of the "Ace Healer" since it can intensify, alter, and relocate vitality. When these quartz gem bowls are used, the organs, tissues, and cells as well as the circulatory, endocrine, and metabolic systems benefit greatly.

The sounds from the gems are heard by the ear, felt throughout the body, invigorates the vagus nerve, and enables vibrations to resound through each concentrated Chakra in the body, resulting in a reasonable and refreshed personality, bodily and spiritual!

Controlling Epilepsy: Vagus Nerve Stimulation

Quantum Brain Healing is based on a foundation of orthomolecular therapies, which include proteins, nutrients, minerals, plants extracts, Chinese natural recipes, and various elective treatments.

Vagus Nerve Stimulation is an option that can be catered for while trying dietary treatment, but it is important to remain open to other options and technologies if this does not meet your goals.

This is a therapeutic gadget that is carefully embedded. Any significant clinic in the US and Europe can embed this gadget for a patient that qualifies.

Vagus Nerve Stimulation (VNS) is a type of neurostimulation that makes an impression on the cerebrum using mild electrical incitement from the vagus nerve in the neck by means of a precisely placed little restorative gadget.

No surgery is necessary for this procedure. Instead, an electric pulse or stimulation is sent by a medical device like a pacemaker to the vagus nerve. The vagus nerve is part of the autonomic nervous system and controls involuntary body functions.

VNS has been affective in controlling epilepsy for patients who haven't had success with epileptic medications or can't tolerate the side effects, and neurosurgery isn't an option.

The embedded restorative device is a small, flat battery that is about the size of a silver dollar in diameter. The VNS medical device was developed by Cyberonics, Inc. The specialist determines the quality and timing of the beats generated by the gadget based on each patient's unique requirements.

The electrical incitement can be adjusted without having to go through surgery again, using a wand that is paired with a computer.

Some of the signs you may experience while receiving VNS treatment include a hoarse voice, coughing, throat pain, trouble breathing, a slight feeling of choking, changes to your voice's pitch or volume,, earache toothache and tingling in the neck.

The implantation site might be susceptible to irritation or illness. VNS has no detrimental impact on the mind. This is a serious medical operation that should not be taken lightly, but it may be a last resort for individuals with uncontrolled epileptic seizures. Consider all alternatives before deciding to stop seizing control.

Did you know that there's a method to help manage anxiety using your vagus nerve? If you're struggling with frequent episodes of anxiety or other related symptoms like nausea, chest pain, and heart palpitations, read on for more information.

By becoming familiar with a basic yet intriguing strategy to control your nervousness by animating your vagus nerve, you'll be able to reduce stress and tension at any time or place - whether that's at home, on the road, or (especially) during uncomfortable work meetings.

Did you know that the FDA approved a vagus nerve stimulator to treat depression by occasionally stimulating the vagus nerve? However, hopefully you won't need surgery. You can experience the benefits of vagus nerve stimulation by learning some simple breathing exercises.

The vagus nerve is the most important part of the parasympathetic nervous system (the one that relaxes you and controls your body's resting response).

The brainstem begins the process, and it "winds" all the way down into the middle of your body, spreading strands to your tongue, pharynx, vocal harmonies, lungs, heart, stomach, digestive organs and proteins that are hostile to stretched (such as Acetylcholine), having an impact on absorption, digestion and obviously the unwinding response.

The vagus nerve helps to connect the mind and body, and is responsible for feelings of compassion and gut instincts. Managing your stress levels and mental state demands the ability to activate the calming anxiety pathways of your parasympathetic nervous system.

While you cannot actively control this part of the nervous system, you can indirectly stimulate your vagus nerve by:

· Drenching your face in cool water (the plunging reflex)

· Endeavoring to breathe out against a shut aviation route (the Valsalva move).

This should be achievable by keeping the mouth shut and pressing the nose while attempting to fill up. The pressure inside the chest pit stimulates the vagus nerve, which causes it to fire.

· Singing

· Inhale with your diaphragm

Obviously, diaphragmatic breathing is more activating. Reinforcing this living sensory system can pay extraordinary benefits, and the best way to accomplish that is by training your breath.

Now is an opportune time to test out this breathing method. The key is to relax your diaphragm and breathe in slowly through your nose. This way of breathing is more natural and beneficial for you overall.

The diaphragm is a primary muscle associated with breathing. Its bell shape allows it to swell out when you inhale and return to cylindrical form when you exhale, thus creating a vacuum that pulls air into your lungs.

When you breathe in properly, it applies pressure downwards against your intestines and other viscera, pushing them gently outward. This is why deep breathing exercises are sometimes called diaphragm breathing or belly relaxation. ↓

· Inhale with the glottis whilst partially shut

When you hold your breath, the glottis is at the back of your tongue and is shut.

By controlling the glottis you are:

a) Controlling the air current, whilst inhaling and exhaling

b) Animating your vagus nerve.

Try this right now

· Synopsis

By learning how to use the vagus nerve to relax, you may assist your body release tension. The vagus nerve acts as the link between your mind and body, and it controls your relaxing response.

You can invigorate your vagus nerve by rehearsing diaphragmatic breathing with the glottis halfway shut. Utilize your dead time to rehearse this system reliably, and you'll be astonished by the outcomes.

The Vagus Nerve and Glossopharyngeal Nerve (Cranial Nerves IX and X) and Their Disorders

The glossopharyngeal and vagus nerves are shown together since they are intimately associated. The glossopharyngeal nerve is made up of a tangible and an engine segment.

The engine filaments emerge from the core in an equivocal pattern, similar to that of the medulla, which is nestled inside the parallel section of the brain. They depart the skull via the jugular foramen along with other nerves and vagus.

The superior and inferior thyroid (th-yoo-rid) branches of the vagus nerve supply the stylopharyngeus muscle, which raises the pharynx. The glossopharyngeal nerve's autonomic efferent filaments originate from the basic salivatory core (sa-li-vai-tor-ree).

Preganglionic filaments go to the otic ganglion through the lesser shallow petrosal nerve. Postganglionic strands then pass through the auriculotemporal (o-ree-kew-low-tem-puh-ruhl) part of the fifth nerve and arrive at the Parotid gland.

The glossopharyngeal nerve's tactile filaments are organized in the petrous ganglion, which is located beneath the jugular foramen and also the unrivaled ganglion, which is tiny.

The exteroceptive filaments supply the pharyngeal tonsils, back mass of the pharynx, and a section of taste sensation on the back third of the tongue. The vagus nerve is longer than any other cranial nerve.

The engine filaments that emerge from the nucleus are ambiguous and supply all of the muscles of the pharynx, along with a sensitive sense of taste and larynx. The exceptions to this are tensor veli palatini and stylopharyngeus.

The parasympathetic filaments are formed in the spinal efferent core and carried to the medulla as preganglionic strands of the craniosacral autonomic sensory system's cranial nerve segment. These fibers terminate at ganglia near the viscera, which they supply via postganglionic filaments.

They function as parasympathetic in action. As a result, vagal incitation leads to bradycardia, bronchial constriction, gastric and pancreatic squeeze discharge, and peristalsis expansion. The tangible component of the vagus is centered in the ganglion and ganglion (nude) on the neck.

The vagus provides sensations from the outer sound-related meatus, pinna and surrounding area, as well as pain sensations from the durometer (a tough protective covering) around the back cranial fossa.

Test the ninth and tenth nerves capacities together as they are usually connected. Ask about symptoms like dysphagia, dysarthria (di-sar-three-uh), liquid spilling from the nose, and a rough voice.

When a patient is forced to open their mouth, the engine component is examined by examining the uvula. The uvula is typically centered. In one-sided vagal loss of motion, the palatal curve becomes straightened and moved down on the same side. On phonation, the uvula veers off to the usual side.

The muffle reflex, or pharyngeal reflex, is set off by placing something like a tongue decompressor or cotton bud on the posterior wall of the throat or tonsil area. When it's working properly, there will be visible movement from the pharyngeal muscles accompanied by tongue withdrawal.

The glossopharyngeal supplies the afferent component of this reflex, whereas the vagus nerve provides the efferent. In either a ninth- or tenth-nerve injury, this reflex is lost. Investigate for general feelings on the back pharyngeal divider, delicate sense of taste and facial tonsils, and taste over the back third of the tongue.

These are impeded in glossopharyngeal loss of motion.

Clutters of ninth and tenth nerve capacities

The occurrence of either nerve being separated is unusual, and they are usually found together; the eleventh and twelfth nerves are frequently impacted. Glossopharyngeal neuralgia (new-rahl-jeeuh), which resembles trigeminal neuralgia, is relatively uncommon.

It starts in the tonsillar fossa with paroxysmal severe agony. It's conceivable that it's linked to bradycardia, and in such circumstances, it's known as vagoglossopharyngeal neuralgia. In most cases, a preliminary of phenytoin or carbamazepine is sufficient to relieve pain.

The motor nerve, sensory fibers, and sympathetic nerves are susceptible to injury as a result of automobile accidents, strokes, or other causes. Vascular sores (such as diabetic ulcers), for example, parallel medullary focal necrosis or bulbar poliomyelitis can produce limb weakness by affecting these nerves simultaneously.

Back fossa tumors and basal meningitis may include damage to these nerves that are outside the cerebrum stem. Complete two-sided vagal loss of motion is incompatible with life. The repetitive laryngeal nerves, particularly the left one, play a role in thoracic sores. This only produces hoarseness of the voice without dysphagia (difficulty swallowing).

Turning Your Vagus On

What are the similarities between nervousness, ruffianism, acid reflux, and restlessness? And you said pressure! When you mentioned absence of pressure, you're in fantastic form! All the more precisely, they are caused by a lack of Vagus activity. Not that kind of Vegas. This sort of Vagus is essential to your health and prosperity.

· Your vagus nerve connects your brain to your heart, stomach, and all of your interior organs. To be honest, its influence is unavoidable to the point that it has been dubbed "the skipper" of your parasympathetic sensory system, which is your body's natural unwind, repair, and restore mechanism.

· Nerve activity is crucial for appropriate functioning of your Vagus nerve, which keeps constant irritation under tight controls and puts the breaks on major sickness. It regulates your heart rate, increasing irregularity, a sign of cardiac health. Furthermore, it warns your lungs to breathe deeply, drawing in fresh oxygen that restores your vital energy.

· Your Vagus nerve doesn't just interpret information from your gut to your brain-- it also gives you "gut feelings" about what is good or bad for you. Then, it helps you connect memories together so that you can recall important information as easily as your best intentions.

· Acetylcholine counters the adrenaline and cortisol secreted in your body during a stress reaction, allowing you to enacted the Relaxation Response and achieve a state of calm.

As a result, you now have an understanding of why actuating your Vagus nerve is so simple. The problem is that our current culture pushes us to be extremely hyper-focused, constantly busy, without realizing it. We're so accustomed to being pushed that we don't know what genuine rest feels like or how to achieve it.

We are always on the move and seldom taking a break. In our society, it is considered taboo to rest or be inactive for long periods of time. We constantly feel guilty if we're not doing something and exhausted when we're not constantly stimulated!

In other words, when we're anxious, irritable, and restless all the time, it prevents us from getting deep rest. This contributes to cancers and other diseases.

Surely regular, slow, deep breathing is extremely important. But there's a problem. Being in a state of constant stress promotes the pattern of restricted, fast, shallow breathing. So, regular slow deep breaths may take some practice to get used to it . Here's an excellent way to do that:

A Simple Deep Breathing Meditation:

Lie on your back and close your eyes. Place one hand over the other on your lower stomach area, just above the navel. As you breathe in, allow your lower abdominal muscles to rise gently with the breath. As you exhale slowly, let those same muscles relax and fall inward toward the spine.

Follow your breath as you sink into a decent easy cadence, daintily following your breath as your stomach gently rises and falls. Consider if it's possible to avoid forcing this to happen while also keeping an eye on it while it happens naturally, effectively, and easily.

As you go, see whether you can identify the moment when you first breathe in and follow it all the way through until you naturally expel. After that, note the minute you begin to breathe out and track it all the way until it naturally stops. Take a few minutes to relax your mind with this soothing rhythm-and then check how wonderful you feel afterward.

Take some time out of your day to try this breathing exercise. You can do it once a day to reduce stress and tension.

You can do this relaxation technique in bed at night before sleep. Soon, you will reset your body's natural balance and live a more peaceful and happy life.

Testing Vagus nerve activity

The Vagus nerve is responsible for our reflex responses like coughing, sneezing, and swallowing. It's key to maintaining good health, so it's important to keep tabs on its state.

Various ways exist that you can use to measure your vagus nerve activity. After learning more about this nervous system and its functions, you have likely come to the realization that this area deserves more attention.

You might want to know where you stand, whether you have a chronic dorsal state or not. The following are some of the ways to assess your vagal nerve activity:

This nerve controls the larynx, pharynx, and uvular muscles, as well as the levator palatini muscles in the back of the throat. This may require assistance from someone else. This approach is very powerful and may change your perspective on your body.

The strongest neural innervations in the neck are also one of the ventral vagus nerve's innervations. The uvula is a teardrop-shaped portion of soft tissue that hangs from the back of your throat down to your chest.

1. Take a flashlight and a friend with you.

2. By examining the inside of their mouth, as well as the back of their neck and uvula, you or a friend can discover if they have strep throat.

3. Ask the person to say "AH."

4. Open your mouth, use a tongue depressor or fingers to push the tongue down so the uvula and soft palate are more visible.

5. You or the examiner can inspect the uvula to discover if it has a deviation.

The difference you are looking for is between one side and the other. If the uvula pulls to one side, it is a sign of a problem with the ventral vagal nerve. However, if it moves up in a symmetrical pattern, you are in a state of social interaction known as the ventral vagal tone - which is generally preferable.

So, for example, if the soft palate only moves up on the left side and not the right, it can be an indication of a problem with the pharyngeal branch of the ventral vagal nerve.

Heart rate variability

This is a method to determine the function of the vagal nerve in research. The ratio between the sympathetic and parasympathetic messages reflects the vagus nerve activity, otherwise known as vagal tone. This aids researchers in understanding how well the vagus nerve is functioning.

The doctor may take an ECG to look for abnormal heart rhythms and assess the heartbeat patterns. Your heart beats faster when you breathe deeply because it is trying to distribute oxygenated blood throughout your body.

The vagus nerve is responsible for the heart's ability to change with its surroundings, otherwise known as heart rate variability (HRV). In general, a lower heart rate and stronger HRV go hand-in-hand with a higher vagal tone.

When your neurological system is performing well and you are socially engaged, there are variations in the time between heartbeats owing to the natural ups and downs of the heart rate in response to breathing, blood pressure, hormones, and emotions.

The difference between these two values is heart rate variability (HRV). High HRV implies a lot of fluctuations in time intervals. HRV may be used as a general health indicator. It's one of the most promising techniques for assessing autonomic nervous system activity.

When the ventral branch of the vagus nerve is functioning properly, heart rate variability is high. A large body of evidence suggests that a high HRV correlates with better health and quality of life.

When the ventral vagus function is diminished, the autonomic nervous system reverts to either a stress state or a dorsal vagal state. Low HRV refers to changes in the time intervals between heartbeats that are less or negligible compared to normal functioning.

In certain investigations, low heart rate variability has been linked to a number of mental problems. HRV, for example, has been found to decrease in response to acute time pressure, post-traumatic stress disorder (PTSD), emotional strain, and increased state anxiety.

Children who have ADHD tend to worry more throughout the day and for longer periods of time, which appears to lower their HRV. Low HRV is also linked with a lack of concentration and motor inhibition.

Low HRV has also been linked to post-traumatic stress disorder. Low HRV is considered to be a sign of poor general health, in terms of physical health, because to low heart rate variability. Obesity, diabetic neuropathy, and the activity of the dorsal vagus nerve are just a few examples of conditions associated with decreased HRV.

For sexual difficulties, some people turn to a doctor or a therapist. Recent study has shed light on women's sexual problems, revealing an association between heart rate variability and these issues.

According to a variety of studies, there is evidence that men are more prone to erectile dysfunction owing to a broader autonomic nervous system imbalance. HRV testing appears to provide useful diagnostic information and can be used as a fast screening method for changes in the autonomic nervous system activity.

If scientific research affirms that the state of the autonomic nervous system plays a role in psychological problems, it may be worthwhile to investigate the possibility of improving heart rate variability and the purpose of the ventral branch of the vagus nerve as a first step in managing psychological issues before relying upon traditional psychological interventions or medication.

The trap and squeeze test

Chronic vagal episodes can result in a lack of muscular tone, particularly in the neck and shoulder. Pain and stiffness are common as a result of this, thus most people seek massage therapy.

The uvula test is more intrusive and takes longer, whereas the palatal palpation test is less so. This may necessitate the assistance of a friend, preferably a healthcare professional such as a physiotherapist, medical practitioner, or competent therapist.

The top of the shoulder is tense, and you just need to squeeze the muscles on top for this test. The Trap Squeeze Test takes only a few seconds and can be used with children and persons on the autistic spectrum, who may typically struggle to offer their cooperation for conventional procedures like as above.

The vagus nerve may be tested by sliding, raising, and rolling the tops of the trapezius muscles on top of the shoulders halfway down to the neck on the left and right sides. Despite its enormous size, the trapezius muscle is quite delicate.

1. Softly squeeze the trapezius muscle on either side between your thumb and first finger. Most beginners merely grip the muscle too tightly; however, it is better to use light pressure.

2. If you squeeze softly and gently, they should be able to raise the muscle somewhat away from the underlying muscles.

3. The skin of the trapezius muscle should be examined. On one hand, they should be able to compare the tonus of the trapezius muscle on the other side to that of their own. Is both sides hard or is one more difficult than the other? Both sides should ideally be soft and stretchy.

Depending on the person, one side is typically soft and elastic while the other isn't. If they were to squeeze gently, they would notice that despite pushing further in, the muscle on one side remains relaxed and malleable. However, the muscle on opposing side may tense up and feel rigid even under mild pressure.

4. The difference in sensation between the two sides is usually when patients realize that something is wrong. It's important to remember that not everyone will describe the feeling differently, but definitive point is that there are different feelings between the left and right side. This may be a sign of vagus nerve dysfunction.

5. Your autonomic nervous system is not socially engaged, meaning you are either experiencing stress or dorsal vagal withdrawal.

The gag-reflex test

A clinician may test the vagus nerve by using the gag reflex. During this test, the doctor will tickle both sides of the back throat with a soft cotton swab. If the person does not gag in response to this stimulation, it could be indicative of a vagus nerve dysfunction.

This is a list of indicators that can assist you in determining where you are with your vagal tone. You may start practicing exercises to stimulate your vagus nerve once you've determined that stimulation is needed.

Causes of Vagus Nerve Damage

Gastroparesis

Gastroparesis is a condition in which the muscles of your stomach (motility) do not function normally. Normally, solid powerful compressions propel food through your gastrointestinal tract.

Be that as it may, in the event that you have gastroparesis, your stomach's motility is reduced or doesn't work by any means, keeping your stomach from discharging appropriately.

Some medicines, like narcotic pain relievers, a few antidepressants, and hypertension and hypersensitivity drugs can cause moderate gastric exhaustion. For people who already have gastroparesis, these prescriptions might make their condition worse.

Gastroparesis can interfere with typical absorption, cause sickness and retching, and create difficulties with glucose levels and nutrition. The source of gastroparesis is typically unknown. It's a result of diabetes in some people, as well as operations.

Despite the fact that there is no cure for gastroparesis, modifications to your diet as well as medicines might assist.

Side effects

Signs and side effects of gastroparesis include:

· Vomiting

· Nausea

· Vomiting undigested nourishment eaten a couple of hours before

- Acid reflux

- Abdominal swelling

- Abdominal pain

- Changes in glucose levels

- Lack of craving

- Weight problems and unhealthiness

Numerous individuals with gastroparesis don't have any recognizable signs and side effects.

Causes

1. Usually, gastroparesis is caused by damage to the vagus nerve, which controls the stomach muscles. However, it's not always clear what causes this damage.

2. The vagus nerve is a sympathetic nerve that controls your stomach's movement and nutrition. It also activates the muscles in your stomach to push food into your tiny digestive system. A damaged vagus nerve usually can't communicate signals to your stomach muscles. This might result in food staying in your tummy for longer rather than going throughout regularly into your little digestive tract to be digested.

3. Sudden or prolonged vagus nerve stimulation can result in damage. The vagus nerve may be damaged by diseases such as diabetes, as well as medical procedures to the stomach and small digestive system.

Hazard factors

Components that can heighten the danger of gastroparesis:

• Diabetes

• Abdominal or esophageal (eh-so-fuh-jee-uhl) medical procedure

• General infection

• Certain medications, such as opiate painkillers, work by slowing the rate at which the stomach empties.

• Scleroderma (skleeuh-ruh-duh-ma) (a connective tissue ailment)

• Nervous system diseases, such as Parkinson's disease or multiple sclerosis

• Hypothyroidism (low thyroid)

Gastroparesis is more common in ladies than it is in males.

Difficulties

Gastroparesis can cause a few difficulties, for example,

• Severe lack of hydration. Continuous spewing can cause lack of hydration.

• When you're malnourished, it's difficult to stay hungry enough to consume the recommended daily caloric intake, or your body might not be able rigorously absorb nutrients due to regurgitation.

• Solidified undigested food that stays in your stomach. Undigested nutrients in your stomach might solidify into a hard lump known as a bezoar. Bezoars can cause nausea and vomiting and may obstruct the passage of nutrients into your small digestive system if they don't get digested.

• Unpredictable glucose changes. Even though gastroparesis isn't linked to diabetes, significant variations in the rate and amount of nutrients delivered into the small intestine can result in erratic glucose levels. These fluctuations in blood sugar level Diabetes is made worse by this. As a consequence, poor glycemic control aggravates gastroparesis.

• Decreased personal satisfaction - An intense eruption of side effects can make it difficult to work and stay focused on different tasks.

Seizure Disorders

When someone has a seizure, their brain's electrical activity is sometimes disrupted, causing some level of temporary mental impairment.

• Many individuals have uncommon sensations just before a seizure begins.

• Although popularized by media, seizures that cause shaking and loss of awareness only occur in a minority of cases. Most often, people simply stop moving or become unaware of their surroundings.

• The source of the conclusion is unknown, but it's likely to be determined by signs. Imaging of the mind, blood testing, and electroencephalography (to record the brain's electrical activity) are usually required to determine the cause.

• If required, medications can for the most part help avert seizures.

The average mind's capacity needs a deliberate, composed, and assisted discharge of electrical driving forces. Electrical incentives give the mind the ability to communicate with the spinal line, nerves, and muscles just as they do within oneself. When the cerebrum's electricity is disrupted, seizures may occur.

Some people may have a seizure at some point in their life, with 66% of those individuals never having another one. Seizure problems usually begin during early adolescence or late adulthood. There are different types of seizures that can occur:

Seizures might be depicted as afflictions:

Epileptic: These seizures don't have a known trigger and they happen multiple times. Epileptic seizures, or a seizure disorder, is called epilepsy. The cause of epileptic seizures is often unknown (idiopathic -epilepsy).

Although migraines might be due to different brain issues, including structural abnormalities, strokes or tumors.

• Epileptic: A non-epileptic seizure is one that is caused by a reversible problem or a condition that affects the brain, such as contamination, stroke, head damage, or reaction to medicine. A fever can cause a non-epileptic seizure in youngsters (known as a febrile (fee-brail) seizure).

Causes

Which illnesses are most prevalent and cause seizures to begin?

• Before age 2: High temperatures or brief metabolic aberrations from the norm, such as high blood sugar (glucose), calcium, magnesium, nutrient B6, or salt levels that are unusual.

The chances of having a seizure are increased if you have a fever or any other variation from the norm. If seizures repeatedly happen without such triggers, it is more likely that damage during birth occurred, resulting in a birth imperfection or an inherited metabolic disorder.

• 2 to 14 years: Often, the reason is obscure (see additionally Seizures in Children).

• Adults: There are many things that can cause a seizure, including head damage, stroke, or tumor. One of the most common reasons for seizures is alcohol withdrawal (when someone abruptly stops drinking). However, for some people in this age group, the exact reason is unknown.

• Older grown-ups: The reason might be a cerebrum tumor or stroke.

Seizures with no recognizable reason are called idiopathic.

Conditions that aggravate the cerebrum, for example, wounds, certain medications, lack of sleep, contaminations, fever—or those that deny the mind of oxygen or fuel, for example, unusual heart rhythms, a low degree of oxygen in the blood, or an extremely low degree of sugar in the blood (hypoglycemia)— can trigger a solitary seizure whether an individual has a seizure issue or not.

A seizure that occurs as a result of this update is referred to as an incited seizure (and, in effect, is a non-epileptic seizure).

Individuals with a seizure issue are bound to have a seizure when they experience the following:

• They are under too much physical or passionate pressure.

• They are inebriated or denied of rest.

• They have abruptly stopped drinking alcohol or taking tranquilizers.

Seizures are caused by a variety of noises, bright lights, computer games, or any other type of contact with specific body parts. Reflex epilepsy is the result of this turmoil.

Diabetes

Diabetics are at risk for neuropathy, which is damage to the nerves. Over time, elevated blood sugar levels can change a nerve's chemical makeup and harm the supportive blood vessels.

Gastroparesis is a condition in which the stomach and intestines are unable to move food effectively through the digestive system, caused by diabetes. Gastroparesis is characterized by nausea, diarrhea, heartburn, constipation, bowel bloating, spasm, and lack of hunger.

Alcoholism

Chronic alcohol abuse, also known as alcoholic neuropathy, involves nerve damage. The autonomic nervous system is damaged by alcohol in a dose-related toxic manner, with the Vagus nerve being affected. Alcohol abstinence will repair the Vagus nerve injury.

Infection and surgical complications

When the vagus nerve is damaged, as it is with upper respiratory viral infections, damage to the nerve can occur. Coughs, nasal blockage and a runny nose are typically indicators of these diseases. In patients who have PVVN symptoms that continue with coughs, throat clearing, communication difficulties, and vocal exhaustion are known as posterior vagal neuropathy or PVVN.

During bariatric surgery, the vagus nerve may be damaged. Damage to the vagus nerve was found in a procedure known as laparoscopic hemic (he-muhk) fundoplication.

Vagus Nerve in medical therapy

Medical science has been researching the medical usage of the vagus nerve since decades, owing to the many vital functions of this nerve.

For decades, the vagotomy procedure (cutting the vagus nerve) was a standard element of therapy for peptic ulcer disease since it reduced stomach acid levels. The vagotomy, on the other hand, has some drawbacks and is now used considerably less frequently owing to the advent of better therapy.

Today, the utilization of electrical stimulators (particularly modified pacemakers) to stimulate the vagus nerve on a constant basis to cure a variety of ailments is quite popular. Vagus nerve stimulators, or VNS devices, have been frequently used in the treatment of severe epilepsy that cannot be controlled with medications. VNS therapy is occasionally used to treat uncontrollable anxiety.

Everything appears like a nail when you have a hammer, so manufacturers of VNS gadgets evaluate their usage in other situations, such as high blood pressure, migraines, tinnitus, fibromyalgia, and weight loss.

VNS technologies are also intriguing. Nonetheless, when the fad dies down, the true potential of VNS will be revealed.

Medical methods and treatments for the Vagus nerve

Vagus Nerve Stimulation

In addition to these criteria, inflammation is a reaction that we all experience in our bodies. Anxiety and inflammatory reactions can be persistent for some people, resulting in additional health issues.

Vagus nerve stimulation is a form of treatment that involves using electrical impulses to stimulate the vagus nerve. This therapy is used for epilepsy and depression cases that have not responded to other forms of treatment.

The unit is usually placed skin-level under the left side of the chest, where a wire attaches it to the vagus nerve. Once activated, signals are sent from the device to your brain stem and then to your brain. The unit is typically controlled by a neurologist but can be magnetically powered for portability by individuals.

Vagus nerve stimulation is believed to not only help with seizures, but multiple sclerosis, Alzheimer's disease, and headaches in the future. If medications don't work to control seizures, this procedure is an option that can be considered.

The Vagus nerve is stimulated by a small electric stimulator placed on the neck near to, but not directly over, the vagus nerve and a power source nearby to the axis or heart. The system works as a cardiac pacemaker for the left vagus nerve. It sends automatic electrical impulses to the brain, which may be triggered manually to prevent seizure onset.

The FDA has approved Vagus nerve stimulation for two separate conditions based on clinical trials that have tested its efficiency.

Epilepsy

The FDA approved the use of Vagus nerve stimulation for unmanageable epilepsy in 1997.

It involves a small electrical tool that is in a person's chest, similar to a pacemaker. A thin wire known as a lead flows to the Vagus nerve from the system.

The system is surgically implanted into the body under general anesthesia. It then sends electrical impulses to the brain via the vagus nerve at regular intervals throughout the day, which reduces or eliminates seizures.

Side effects of the Vagus nerve stimulation include:

· Sort throat

· Change in voice

· Coughing

· Shortness of breath

· Difficulty swallowing

· Nausea or stomach discomfort

Patients must always inform their doctor if they have any concerns regarding the medication, as there may be ways to lower or prevent epileptic seizures.

Who Can Benefit From This Stimulation

Vagus nerve stimulation may help patients with intractable epilepsy who have uncontrollable seizures or loss of consciousness during complex partial epileptic episodes or general convulsions.

Epilepsy medications may reduce or eliminate epileptic fits, although not everyone will notice a difference. In all situations, the patient must continue taking anti-epileptic medicines before using the stimulator. Some months after inserting a vagal nerve stimulator, the neurologist may recommend that the patient take a lower dose of medicine.

Evaluation

A vagal nerve stimulator will not be inserted until the doctor has done a complete assessment of the patient's medical condition. The doctor will go through the patient's medical record, inquire about their personal medical history and that of their family.

All medications the patient has taken, including electronic drugs, vitamins, nutritional supplements and herbal remedies should be recorded in the data. All medicines are accessible.

Procedure

The vagal nerve stimulator is a device implanted during an operation that takes one to two hours. The stimulator, which comprises of a battery and wire, is attached to a nerve in the neck and programmed to periodically activate it. typically needs its batteries replaced every 10 years; however, this can be achieved with local anesthesia during a simple procedure that does not require hospitalization.

During the pulsation, some people may experience tingling or a hoarse voice; nevertheless, with time, most individuals get used to these sensations. The doctors make sure that the vagal nerve stimulator is working correctly and assists in seizure management.

The benefits of VNS may be:

• Having less severe seizures

- Having fewer seizures

- Having enhanced quality of life

- Possibly less epileptic medication

If you have a VNS device fitted, you will probably find that your emergency management improves slowly over time. Six out of ten people with a fitted VNS feel that their number of seizures is halved. However, problems do still occur in between three and six percent of people with VNS devices. These were generally due to issues with the device itself and sorted by having a second operation.

Why should you be careful if you Have VNS

MRI scans

It's critical for all participants to understand the VNS system in case you're advised to have an MRI. You may need to take precautions to ensure that the scan is conducted in a secure manner. To provide evidence of your diagnosis, you should carry with you a neurologist patient MRI form.

Airport security scanners

The airport's security systems should not be affected or harmed by the safety sensors. VNS Therapy device makers recommend that you show your VNS Therapy ID card to airport security in order to be safe; otherwise, you may get a pat-down search.

Certain devices that detect when they are close to other types of equipment will affect your generator.

• The doctor will provide you with guidance on warning signs to look for that indicate it is no longer safe for you to wear a pacemaker. This is because equipment that may affect your pacemaker, may also influence your VNS generator.

• Maintain a distance of 60 centimetres or 2 feet from shop deactivators of Electronic Article Surveillance System labels to prevent your generator from being tripped. The deactivators are generally located near store entrances.

• Tablets, vibrators, and other electronic devices can emit electromagnetic fields that you should keep at least 20 cm or 8 inches away from your chest. If you notice any discomfort while using these devices, move away from the device or switch it off to alleviate the problem.

Vagus Nerve Stimulation Techniques - Probiotics

The 'gut-brain axis' is the relationship between the gastrointestinal system and the central nervous system. It is now seen as a possible avenue for treatment of disorders that affect the Central Nervous System because it has been increasingly looked upon as a symbiotic relationship inthe body.

The gut-brain axis is the relationship between the gastrointestinal tract and the brain. This approach can help solve many health problems associated with a breakdown in communication between these two systems. By manipulating microbiotics and probiotics, we can treat and prevent diseases that have been linked to problems with the nervous system.

Gastrointestinal health and CNS disorders, like ASD, are obviously linked. This connection makes the manipulation process--a treatment where you physically move someone's body parts around to ease pain or help with movement--relevant for treating these conditions. Health care practitioners are increasingly using this method because it is effective in addressing some problems their patients experience through the Central Nervous System.

This type of therapy aims to repair the neurological pathways in the central nervous system that have been disrupted due to disease. Over the past decade, there has been an increase in evidence linking host-microbe interactions at all levels of complexity, from direct cell-to-cell communication to widespread systemic signaling, and impacting a wide range of organs and organ systems, including the central nervous system.

This treatment approach is key to pick the best possible way of implementing a relevant cure for the central nervous system. Probiotics are an essential part of any diet and can be helpful for many problems from digestive issues to skin conditions. Additionally, probiotics might also help in promoting the vagus nerve."

A 2011 scientific study found that when mice were given Lactobacillus Rhamnosus, it increased their GABA production and relieved tension, anxiety, as well as habits related to anxiety.

What are probiotics?

Probiotics are live germs and yeasts that are beneficial to your gastrointestinal system. Due to their role in maintaining your gut health, probiotics are often known as "wonderful" or "useful" germs.

Probiotics can be found in pills and some food items, such as yogurt. They're typically given to assist with digestion issues.

How Do They Work?

Scientists are looking to figure out how probiotics function. Probiotics may help to transform "great" germs in your body, such as those that you acquire after taking prescription antibiotics.

They can assist in stabilizing your "good" and "bad" germs to keep your body working the way it should.

Kinds of Probiotics

There are many types of germs that can be classified as probiotics, and each one offers different benefits. However, most come from two groups. Talk to your doctor about which one would be best for you.

Bifidobacteria (bai-fi-doh-bacteria) is one of the most common probiotics. It can help with diarrhea and might be able to assist people who are lactose intolerant. You can find it in some dairy products or as a supplement. It might also help relieve the symptoms of irritable bowel syndrome (IBS).

Saccharomyces (sakoh-roh-mai-sees) boulardii is a yeast found in probiotics. This yeast may help reduce symptoms of diarrhea and other digestive problems.

What Do They Do?

Probiotics, for example, aid in the transmission of food through your gut by affecting nerves that control gut movement. Researchers are still researching which probiotics are ideal for specific diseases. Some typical conditions they deal with are:

· Irritable bowel syndrome

· Inflammatory bowel illness (IBD)

· Transmittable diarrhea (triggered by parasites, infections, or germs)

· Diarrhea triggered by prescription antibiotics

Some studies have also shown that they can help with issues in other regions of your body. Some individuals state they have actually assisted with:

· Skin conditions, like eczema.

· Vaginal and urinary health.

· Preventing colds and allergic reactions.

· Oral health.

Probiotics and the Vagus Nerve for Psychiatric Conditions

The vagus nerve is responsible for the regulation of the parasympathetic nervous system. This means that the vagus nerve can play a role in different mental disorders such as anxiety, stress, and post-traumatic syndrome disorder (PTSD). These conditions are often linked to gastrointestinal issues and inflammation.

VNS may be effectively utilized to alleviate anxiety. Several observational research papers have identified that VNS is a reliable and safe therapy for psychiatric problems like anxiety. According on the results of a European multicenter study, vagal nerve stimulation resulted in "an action rate of 37% and a remissions rate of 17%. In treatment-resistant individuals with anxiety, the reaction rate increased to 53% after one year of therapy, while the remission rate rose to 33%.

The pathophysiology of anxiety consists of an inefficient HPA axis, swelling, and imbalances with monoamine transmission. These can all be controlled by vagal activity. Vagal nerve stimulation can help to regulate monoamine metabolism by raising the levels of dopamine, norepinephrine, and serotonin in the body. This lowers corticotropin levels and helps to regulate the HPA axis.

These favorable interactions between lactic acid germs in the brain and the gut happen just by means of the vagus nerve.

In another study, the probiotic Bifidobacteria longum was administered and resulted in anxiolytic impacts. However, these results depended on vagal nerve stability, suggesting its function as an arbitrator between microbiota and psychiatric conditions.

The target of afferent neurons in the vagus nerve are impacted by neuroactive germs, such as L. rhamnosus and B. longum, which send messages from the microbes to the brain. The healthy microbiota produces great quantities of short-chain fats, for example butyric acid, that directly trigger efferent vagal terminals to send messages from the gut to the brain.

Polysaccharides are not to be the only requirement for bacterial vagal nerve stimulation, as lipids play a role too. This is illustrated with B. fragilis (fra-juh-lis), which does not require lipids for activation of Vagal afferent neurons.

Tolllike receptor 4s (TLR4) are located on vagal efferent fibers, and they can detect items such as LPS(lipopolysaccharides) from bacteria to set off both the afferent fibers and brain cells.

The interest in how professionals may enhance vagal activity as a potential alternative to numerous popular psychiatric diseases is shifting toward how specialists may increase vagal function as a basic therapy. We are starting to comprehend that the microbiome might be the target for enhancing vagal activity, and thus, enhancing anxiety, stress and anxiety and other typical psychiatric conditions.

Health Benefits of Taking Probiotics

Probiotics can assist food digestion.

More and more clinical evidence is surfacing that suggests you can manage, and even prevent certain diseases by consuming specific live germs through supplements and food. People in Northern Europe consume probiotics, which come from fermented foods like yogurt, more often than other people because it is part of their culture.

Some experts in the field of digestion argue that probiotic supplements can be helpful for conditions where standard medication falls short, such as irritable bowel syndrome. In the 1990s, medical studies showed that probiotics could help with various gut disorders, prevent allergies in children, and treat urinary tract infections and other problems in women.

Self-medication with germs may not be as extravagant as it appears. Gut microorganisms keep pathogenic bacteria in check, assist with meal digestion and absorption of nutrients, and aid in the immune system's function.

Advantages of Taking Probiotics

Not all probiotics are created equal. Different strains of bacteria react differently to various stimuli. For example, one might be effective in combating cavity-causing organisms in our mouths and doesn't need to survive the journey through our digestive system to work.

According to research, these friendly animals have many potential health benefits. Probiotics have been shown to improve or prevent:

· Diarrhea.

· Irritable bowel syndrome.

· Ulcerative colitis.

· Crohn's illness.

· H. pylori (the reason for ulcers).

· Vaginal infections.

· Urinary system infections.

· Reoccurrence of bladder cancer.

· Infection of the gastrointestinal system triggered by Clostridium difficile.

· Pouchitis (a possible negative effects of surgical treatment that gets rid of the colon).

· Eczema in kids.

Probiotics and gut health.

The most successful probiotic treatment has been for diarrhea. Clinical trials have shown that Lactobacillus GG can shorten the duration of infectious diarrhea in children and infants (but not adults). Probiotics are used to treat a variety of ailments, yet there is little research on the effectiveness and safety of these products. Probiotic supplements have not been proven safe or effective in clinical trials for children less than three years old. However, investigations into probiotics' effects on other health problems are limited since they are mostly restricted and information is unavailable. When compared with a placebo, probiotic pills reduced antibiotic-associated diarrhea by 60% in two large studies.

Diarrhea is the most frequent medical condition, but irregularity is not. The absence of feces in your rectum or anus is unusual; it's known as constipation. Constipation, on the other hand, may be treated with probiotics in a number of different ways: For example, they improve the variety of weekly defecation by 1.3, and they decrease gut transit time by 12.4 hours - compared to standard therapy - which makes passing stools much easier than normal treatment would produce them. The jury is still out on particular suggestions when it comes to the advantages of probiotics for irregularity.

However, numerous little research studies suggest that particular probiotics may aid in the maintenance of ulcerative colitis remission and prevent Crohn's disease relapse and pouchitis (a surgical treatment problem).

Various people are taking probiotics since there is so much evidence for the specific stress they're dealing with, due to all the proof that exists for these circumstances.

Probiotics and Vaginal Health

Probiotics might also help with urinary health. Probiotic therapy that restores the microflora balance may be useful for such standard female urogenital problems as bacterial vaginosis, yeast infection, and urinary tract infection.

Many women eat yogurt or insert it into their vaginas to treat recurring yeast infections, even though medical science does not support this "folk" treatment very much. Researchers are still studying whether probiotics can help treat urinary tract infections.

While probiotics are typically safe, as they exist in a typical gastrointestinal system-- there is always a theoretical risk for individuals with impaired immune function. Always double-check that the Probiotic ingredients are plainly marked on the label and familiar to you or your health supplier. There is no way to test unknown mixes for safety purposes.

Probiotic Supplements

In the United States, a lot of probiotics are sold as dietary supplements, which do not go through the same screening and approval process that pharmaceuticals do. The health benefits of specific strains change from one circumstance to the next, so you might wish to consult a professional who is knowledgeable about probiotics before making any decisions.

CONCLUSION

If you want to start the journey of self-healing, it all starts with you and your willingness to improve your spiritual, mental, emotional, and physical health. A new approach that is recently becoming popular for fighting disease and combating illness is via vagus nerve stimulation. The vagus nerve has a profound influence on our brain's wiring, which in turn can positively affect different aspects of our health.

The vagus nerve is one example of how we can use our bodies to achieve a more balanced life. The exercises, tips and tricks in this book are designed to help you identify areas of your life that might need improvement and provide guidance on how to make those changes.

The great thing about the techniques described in this book is that they may be done at home in your own time and without the need for expensive medications or therapies. Although self-healing might not cure illness, it can help you better understand your medical condition and make you more comfortable with finding holistic methods to aid manage a specific and concerning malady.

It's crucial to understand that in order for healing to take place, it must originate from the inside out before the outside can be healed. There are a lot of expectations for the future concerning this nerve and how it may heal illnesses and minimize disease susceptibility. It is critical to follow through with the exercises described above until they become something you do automatically.

I'd like to extend my sincerest thanks for investing the time to read through this book. I truly hope that it had a beneficial influence on your life or way of thinking.

The vagus nerve is a superhighway between your body and brain, as we discuss in yoga. Its five branches carry information between the two organs, with four of them transporting data from the body to the brain and one transporting data from the brain to the body.

This is the most apparent physical manifestation of the link between mind and body. The Vagus nerve also perceives and regulates the interior world (through its sensory neurons and motor neurons). Because much of the nerve's activity is determined by how information is transferred, we can now split incoming information into two categories: body-to-brain and brain-to-body.

The Vagus nerve has many responsibilities, some which we have known about for a long time, and others which are relatively new discoveries. And there is still more to learn; currently, electrical stimulation of the Vagus nerve is being used as treatment for conditions such as autism, rheumatoid arthritis, and depression.

Healthy Recipes for Vagus Nerve

Chili-lime Cucumber, Jicama, & Apple Sticks

Servings: 3

Cooking Time: 10 Minutes

Ingredients:

- 6 spears cucumber
- 6 spears very ripe apple
- 6 spears jicama (you can use mango instead)
- 1 teaspoon chili lime seasoning
- 2 lime wedges

Directions:

1. In a bowl, mix together cucumber, apple, jicama, lime juice, chili lime seasoning until well combined. Serve garnished with lime wedges. Enjoy!

Nutrition:

324 Calories 24g fat 20g protein 7g carbs

Sardine Meatballs

Servings:3

Cooking Time:10 Minutes

Ingredients:

- 11 oz sardines, canned, drained
- 1/3 cup shallot, chopped
- 1 teaspoon chili flakes
- ½ teaspoon salt
- 2 tablespoon wheat flour, whole grain
- 1 egg, beaten
- 1 tablespoon chives, chopped
- 1 teaspoon olive oil
- 1 teaspoon butter

Directions:

1. Put the butter in the skillet and melt it.
2. Add shallot and cook it until translucent.
3. After this, transfer the shallot in the mixing bowl.
4. Add sardines, chili flakes, salt, flour, egg, chives, and mix up until smooth with the help of the fork.
5. Make the medium size cakes and place them in the skillet.
6. Add olive oil.
7. Roast the fish cakes for 3 minutes from each side over the medium heat.
8. Dry the cooked fish cakes with the paper towel if needed and transfer in the serving plates.

Nutrition:

calories 221, fat 12.2, fiber 0.1, carbs 5.4, protein 21.3

Homemade Salsa

Servings:8

Cooking Time:30 Minutes

Ingredients:

- 12 oz grape tomatoes, halved
- 1/4 cup fresh cilantro, chopped
- 1 fresh lime juice
- 28 oz tomatoes, crushed
- 1 tbsp garlic, minced
- 1 green bell pepper, chopped
- 1 red bell pepper, chopped
- 2 onions, chopped
- 6 whole tomatoes
- Salt

Directions:

1. Add whole tomatoes into the instant pot and gently smash the tomatoes.
2. Add remaining ingredients except cilantro, lime juice, and salt and stir well.
3. Seal pot with lid and cook on high for 5 minutes.
4. Once done, allow to release pressure naturally for 10 minutes then release remaining using quick release. Remove lid.
5. Add cilantro, lime juice, and salt and stir well.
6. Serve and enjoy.

Nutrition:

Calories 146 Fat 1.2 g Carbohydrates 33.2 g Sugar 4 g Protein 6.9 g Cholesterol 0 mg

Kale Chips

Servings: 3

Cooking Time: 5 Minutes

Ingredients:

- 1 lb. fresh kale leaves, stemmed and torn
- ¼ tsp. cayenne pepper
- Salt, to taste
- 1 tbs. olive oil

Directions:

1. Preheat the oven to 350 degrees F. Line a large baking sheet with a parchment paper.
2. Place the kale pieces onto preparation ared baking sheet in a single layer.
3. Sprinkle the kale with cayenne and salt and drizzle with oil.
4. Bake for about 10-15 minutes.

Nutrition:

242 Calories 25g carbs 12g fat 13g protein

Feta Tomato Sea Bass

Servings:3

Cooking Time:8 Minutes

Ingredients:

- 4 sea bass fillets
- 1 1/2 cups water
- 1 tbsp olive oil
- 1 tsp garlic, minced
- 1 tsp basil, chopped
- 1 tsp parsley, chopped
- 1/2 cup feta cheese, crumbled
- 1 cup can tomatoes, diced
- Pepper
- Salt

Directions:

1. Season fish fillets with pepper and salt.
2. Pour 2 cups of water into the instant pot then place steamer rack in the pot.
3. Place fish fillets on steamer rack in the pot.
4. Seal pot with lid and cook on high for 5 minutes.
5. Once done, release pressure using quick release. Remove lid.
6. Remove fish fillets from the pot and clean the pot.
7. Add oil into the inner pot of instant pot and set the pot on sauté mode.
8. Add garlic and sauté for 1 minute.
9. Add tomatoes, parsley, and basil and stir well and cook for 1 minute.
10. Add fish fillets and top with crumbled cheese and cook for a minute.
11. Serve and enjoy

Nutrition:

Calories 219 Fat 10.1 g Carbohydrates 4 g Sugar 2.8 g Protein 27.1 g Cholesterol 70 mg

Crab Stew

Servings:2

Cooking Time:13 Minutes

Ingredients:

- 1/2 lb lump crab meat
- 2 tbsp heavy cream
- 1 tbsp olive oil
- 2 cups fish stock
- 1/2 lb shrimp, shelled and chopped
- 1 celery stalk, chopped
- 1/2 tsp garlic, chopped
- 1/4 onion, chopped
- Pepper
- Salt

Directions:

1. Add oil into the inner pot of instant pot and set the pot on sauté mode.
2. Add onion and sauté for 3 minutes.
3. Add garlic and sauté for 30 seconds.
4. Add remaining ingredients except for heavy cream and stir well.
5. Seal pot with lid and cook on high for 10 minutes.
6. Once done, release pressure using quick release. Remove lid.
7. Stir in heavy cream and serve

Nutrition:

Calories 376 Fat 25.5 g Carbohydrates 5.8 g Sugar 0.7 g Protein 48.1 g Cholesterol 326 mg

Trail Mix

Servings: 3

Cooking Time: 10 Minutes

Ingredients:

- ¼ cup unsalted roasted peanuts
- ¼ cup whole shelled almonds
- ¼ cup chopped pitted dates
- ¼ cup dried cranberries
- 2 ounces dried apricots

Directions:

1. In a medium bowl, mix together all the ingredients until well combined. Enjoy!

Nutrition:

448 Calories 27g fat 41g carbs 15g protein

Berry & Veggie Gazpacho

Servings: 3

Cooking Time: 30 Minutes

Ingredients:

- 1½ lb. fresh strawberries, hulled and sliced
- ½ C. red bell pepper, seeded and chopped
- 1 small cucumber, peeled, seeded and chopped
- ¼ C. onion, chopped
- ¼ C. fresh basil leaves
- 1 small garlic clove, chopped
- ¼ of small jalapeño pepper, seeded and chopped
- 1 tbsp. olive oil
- 3 tbsp. balsamic vinegar

Directions:

1. In a high-speed blender, add all ingredients and pulse until smooth.
2. Transfer the gazpacho into a large bowl.
3. Cover and refrigerate to chill completely before serving.

Nutrition:

448 Calories 27g fat 41g carbs 15g protein

Meat-filled Phyllo (samboosek)

Servings:1

Cooking Time:10 Minutes

Ingredients:

- 1 lb. ground beef or lamb
- 1 medium yellow onion, finely chopped
- 1 TB. seven spices
- 1 tsp. salt
- 1 pkg. frozen phyllo dough (12 sheets)
- 2/3 cup butter, melted

Directions:

1. In a medium skillet over medium heat, brown beef for 3 minutes, breaking up chunks with a wooden spoon.
2. Add yellow onion, seven spices, and salt, and cook for 5 to 7 minutes or until beef is browned and onions are translucent. Set aside, and let cool.
3. Place first sheet of phyllo on your work surface, brush with melted butter, lay second sheet of phyllo on top, and brush with melted butter. Cut sheets into 3-inch-wide strips.
4. Spoon 2 tablespoons meat filling at end of each strip, and fold end strip to cover meat and form a triangle. Fold pointed end up and over to the opposite end, and you should see a triangle forming. Continue to fold up and then over until you come to the end of strip.
5. Place phyllo pies on a baking sheet, seal side down, and brush tops with butter. Repeat with remaining phyllo and filling.
6. Bake for 10 minutes or until golden brown.
7. Remove from the oven and set aside for 5 minutes before serving warm or at room temperature

Nutrition:

242 Calories 25g carbs 12g fat 13g protein

Raw Turmeric Cashew Nut & Coconut Balls

Servings: 3

Cooking Time: 10 Minutes

Ingredients:

- 1 cup raw cashews
- 1 1/2 cup shredded coconut
- 1 tablespoon raw honey
- 3 teaspoons ground turmeric
- 1 teaspoon cinnamon
- 1 teaspoon ground ginger
- 1 teaspoon black pepper
- 1/2 teaspoon sea salt

Directions:

1. In a food processor, process coconut until almost oily; add in the rest of the ingredients and process until cashews are finely chopped.
2. Press the mixture into bite-sized balls and arrange them on a baking tray. Refrigerate until firm before serving

Nutrition:

324 Calories 24g fat 20g protein 7g carbs

Ginger Tahini Dip With Veggies

Servings:3

Cooking Time:10 Minutes

Ingredients:

- ½ cup tahini
- 1 teaspoon grated garlic
- 2 teaspoons ground turmeric
- 1 tablespoon grated fresh ginger
- ¼ cup apple cider vinegar
- ¼ cup water
- ½ teaspoon salt

Directions:

1. In a bowl, whisk together tahini, turmeric, ginger, water, vinegar, garlic, and salt until well blended. Serve with assorted veggies

Nutrition:

448 Calories 27g fat 41g carbs 15g protein

Crunchy Veggie Chips

Servings:3

Cooking Time:17 Minutes

Ingredients:

- 1 cup thinly sliced portobello mushrooms
- 1 cup thinly sliced zucchini
- 1 cup thinly sliced sweet potatoes
- 1 tablespoon extra-virgin olive oil
- Pinch of sea salt
- Pinch of pepper

Directions:

1. Place veggies in a baking dish and drizzle with olive oil; sprinkle with salt and pepper and toss to coat well; bake at 325°F for about 12 minutes or until crunchy. Enjoy!

Nutrition:

448 Calories 27g fat 41g carbs 15g protein

Honey Garlic Shrimp

Servings:3

Cooking Time: 5 Minutes

Ingredients:

- 1 lb shrimp, peeled and deveined
- 1/4 cup honey
- 1 tbsp garlic, minced
- 1 tbsp ginger, minced
- 1 tbsp olive oil
- 1/4 cup fish stock
- Pepper
- Salt

Directions:

1. Add shrimp into the large bowl. Add remaining ingredients over shrimp and toss well.
2. Transfer shrimp into the instant pot and stir well.
3. Seal pot with lid and cook on high for 5 minutes.
4. Once done, release pressure using quick release. Remove lid.
5. Serve and enjoy.

Nutrition:

Calories 240 Fat 5.6 g Carbohydrates 20.9 g Sugar 17.5 g Protein 26.5 g Cholesterol 239 mg

Pita Chips

Servings: 3

Cooking Time: 30 Minutes

Ingredients:

- 6 whole wheat pitas, cut each into 8 wedges
- 2 tsp. olive oil
- Red chili powder, to taste
- Garlic powder, to taste
- Pinch of salt

Directions:

1. Preheat the oven to 400 degrees F.
2. In the bottom of a large baking sheet, place the pita wedges.
3. Brush the both sides of each with oil and sprinkle with chili powder, garlic powder and salt.
4. Now, arrange the pita wedges in a single layer.
5. Bake for about 8 minutes or until golden brown.
6. Serve with your favorite dip

Nutrition:

242 Calories 25g carbs 12g fat 13g protein

Leeks And Calamari Mix

Servings:6

Cooking Time:15 Minutes

Ingredients:

- 2 tablespoon avocado oil
- 2 leeks, chopped
- 1 red onion, chopped
- Salt and black to the taste
- 1 pound calamari rings
- 1 tablespoon parsley, chopped
- 1 tablespoon chives, chopped
- 2 tablespoons tomato paste

Directions:

1. Heat up a pan with the avocado oil over medium heat, add the leeks and the onion, stir and sauté for 5 minutes.
2. Add the rest of the ingredients, toss, simmer over medium heat for 10 minutes, divide into bowls and serve

Nutrition:

calories 238, fat 9, fiber 5.6, carbs 14.4, protein 8.4

Cucumber Rolls

Servings:3

Cooking Time:10 Minutes

Ingredients:

- 1 big cucumber, sliced lengthwise
- 1 tablespoon parsley, chopped
- 8 ounces canned tuna, drained and mashed
- Salt and black pepper to the taste
- 1 teaspoon lime juice

Directions:

1. Arrange cucumber slices on a working surface, divide the rest of the ingredients, and roll.
2. Arrange all the rolls on a platter and serve as an appetizer.

Nutrition:

calories 200, fat 6, fiber 3.4, carbs 7.6, protein 3.5

Parmesan Chips

Servings:4

Cooking Time:20 Minutes

Ingredients:

- 1 zucchini
- 2 oz Parmesan, grated
- ½ teaspoon paprika
- 1 teaspoon olive oil

Directions:

1. Trim zucchini and slice it into the chips with the help of the vegetable slices.
2. Then mix up together Parmesan and paprika.
3. Sprinkle the zucchini chips with olive oil.
4. After this, dip every zucchini slice in the cheese mixture.
5. Place the zucchini chips in the lined baking tray and bake for 20 minutes at 375F.
6. Flip the zucchini sliced onto another side after 10 minutes of cooking.
7. Chill the cooked chips well.

Nutrition:

calories 64, fat 4.3, fiber 0.6, carbs 2.3, protein 5.2

Grape, Celery & Parsley Reviver

Servings:2

Cooking Time:10 Minutes

Ingredients:

- 75g 3ozred grapes
- 3 sticks of celery
- 1 avocado, de-stoned and peeled
- 1 tablespoon fresh parsley
- ½ teaspoon matcha powder

Directions:

1. Place all of the ingredients into a blender with enough water to cover them and blitz until smooth and creamy. Add crushed ice to make it even more refreshing.

Nutrition:

Calories 334 ,Fat 1.5 g ,Carbohydrate 42.9 g ,Protein 6 g

Tomato Triangles

Servings:6

Cooking Time: 10 Minutes

Ingredients:

- 6 corn tortillas
- 1 tablespoon cream cheese
- 1 tablespoon ricotta cheese
- ½ teaspoon minced garlic
- 1 tablespoon fresh dill, chopped
- 2 tomatoes, sliced

Directions:

1. Cut every tortilla into 2 triangles.
2. Then mix up together cream cheese, ricotta cheese, minced garlic, and dill.
3. Spread 6 triangles with cream cheese mixture.
4. Then place sliced tomato on them and cover with remaining tortilla triangles.

Nutrition:

calories 71, fat 1.6, fiber 2.1, carbs 12.8, protein 2.3

Asparagus Frittata

Servings:4

Cooking Time:15 Minutes

Ingredients:

- ¼ cup onion, chopped
- Drizzle of olive oil
- 1-pound asparagus spears, cut into 1-inch pieces
- Salt and ground black pepper to taste
- 4 eggs, whisked
- 1 cup cheddar cheese, grated

Directions:

1. Heat a pan with the oil over medium-high heat, add the onions, stir, and cook for 3 minutes. Add the asparagus, stir, and cook for 6 minutes. Add the eggs, stir, and cook for 3 minutes.
2. Add the salt and pepper sprinkle with the cheese, put in an oven, and broil for 3 minutes.
3. Divide the frittata onto plates and serve.

Nutrition:

Calories 200 ,Fat 12 g ,Carbs 5 g ,Protein 14 g

Salmon And Broccoli

Servings:3

Cooking Time:20 Minutes

Ingredients:

- 2 tablespoons balsamic vinegar
- 1 broccoli head, florets separated
- 4 pieces salmon fillets, skinless
- 1 big red onion, roughly chopped
- 1 tablespoon olive oil
- Sea salt and black pepper to the taste

Directions:

1. In a baking dish, combine the salmon with the broccoli and the rest of the ingredients, introduce in the oven and bake at 390 degrees F for 20 minutes.
2. Divide the mix between plates and serve.

Nutrition:

calories 302, fat 15.5, fiber 8.5, carbs 18.9, protein 19.8

Chili Mango And Watermelon Salsa

Servings:8

Cooking Time:10 Minutes

Ingredients:

- 1 red tomato, chopped
- Salt and black pepper to the taste
- 1 cup watermelon, seedless, peeled and cubed
- 1 red onion, chopped
- 2 mangos, peeled and chopped
- 2 chili peppers, chopped
- ¼ cup cilantro, chopped
- 3 tablespoons lime juice
- Pita chips for serving

Directions:

1. In a bowl, mix the tomato with the watermelon, the onion and the rest of the ingredients except the pita chips and toss well.
2. Divide the mix into small cups and serve with pita chips on the side.

Nutrition:

calories 62, fat 4.7, fiber 1.3, carbs 3.9, protein 2.3

Chia Crackers

Servings: 24

Cooking Time:

Ingredients:

- 1/2 cup pecans, chopped
- 1/2 cup chia seeds
- 1/2 tsp. cayenne pepper
- 1 cup water
- 1/4 cup nutritional yeast
- 1/2 cup pumpkin seeds
- 1/4 cup ground flax
- Salt and pepper, to taste

Directions:

1. Mix around 1/2 cup of chia seeds and 1 cup of water. Keep it aside.
2. Take another bowl and combine all the remaining ingredients. Combine well and stir in the chia water mixture until you obtained dough.
3. Transfer the dough onto a baking sheet and roll it out into a ¼"-thick dough.
4. Transfer into a preheated oven at 325°F and bake for about ½ hour.
5. Take out from the oven, flip over the dough, and cut it into desired cracker shaped-squares.
6. Spread and back again for a further half an hour, or until crispy and browned.
7. Once done, take them out from the oven and let them cool at room temperature. Enjoy!

Nutrition:

Calories: 41 ,Fats: 3.1 g ,Carbs: 2 g ,Protein: 2 g

Pepper Salmon Skewers

Servings:5

Cooking Time:15 Minutes

Ingredients:

- 1.5-pound salmon fillet
- ½ cup Plain yogurt
- 1 teaspoon paprika
- 1 teaspoon turmeric
- 1 teaspoon red pepper
- 1 teaspoon salt
- 1 teaspoon dried cilantro
- 1 teaspoon sunflower oil
- ½ teaspoon ground nutmeg

Directions:

1. For the marinade: mix up together Plain yogurt, paprika, turmeric red pepper, salt, and ground nutmeg.
2. Chop the salmon fillet roughly and put it in the yogurt mixture.
3. Mix up well and marinate for 25 minutes.
4. Then skew the fish on the skewers.
5. Sprinkle the skewers with sunflower oil and place in the tray.
6. Bake the salmon skewers for 15 minutes at 375F.

Nutrition:

calories 217, fat 9.9, fiber 0.6, carbs 4.2, protein 28.1

Garlic Mussels

Servings: 4

Cooking Time: 10 Minutes

Ingredients:

- 1-pound mussels
- 1 chili pepper, chopped
- 1 cup chicken stock
- ½ cup milk
- 1 teaspoon olive oil
- 1 teaspoon minced garlic
- 1 teaspoon ground coriander
- ½ teaspoon salt
- 1 cup fresh parsley, chopped
- 4 tablespoons lemon juice

Directions:

1. Pour milk in the saucepan.
2. Add chili pepper, chicken stock, olive oil, minced garlic, ground coriander, salt, and lemon juice.
3. Bring the liquid to boil and add mussels.
4. Boil the mussel for 4 minutes or until they will open shells.
5. Then add chopped parsley and mix up the meal well.
6. Remove it from the heat

Nutrition:

calories 136, fat 4.7, fiber 0.6, carbs 7.5, protein 15.3

Superfood Spiced Apricot-sesame Bliss Balls

Servings: 3

Cooking Time: 30 Minutes

Ingredients:

- 2 tablespoons sesame seeds
- 1 cup apricots
- 1 cup natural gluten-free muesli
- 1 cup almonds
- 2 tablespoons raw honey
- 1 teaspoon ground cinnamon

Directions:

- In a food processor, process almonds until finely chopped; add in raw honey, muesli, apricots, and cinnamon and process until very smooth.
- Add sesame seeds in a shallow dish. Roll two tablespoons of the almond mixture into bite-sized balls and then roll them into the sesame seeds until well coated.
- Arrange them on a tray and refrigerate until set. Serve and store the rest in an airtight container.

Nutrition:

448 Calories 27g fat 41g carbs 15g protein

Halibut And Quinoa Mix

Servings:4

Cooking Time:30 Minutes

Ingredients:

- 4 halibut fillets, boneless
- 2 tablespoons olive oil
- 1 teaspoon rosemary, dried
- 2 teaspoons cumin, ground
- 1 tablespoons coriander, ground
- 2 teaspoons cinnamon powder
- 2 teaspoons oregano, dried
- A pinch of salt and black pepper
- 2 cups quinoa, cooked
- 1 cup cherry tomatoes, halved
- 1 avocado, peeled, pitted and sliced
- 1 cucumber, cubed
- ½ cup black olives, pitted and sliced
- Juice of 1 lemon

Directions:

- In a bowl, combine the fish with the rosemary, cumin, coriander, cinnamon, oregano, salt and pepper and toss.
- Heat up a pan with the oil over medium heat, add the fish, and sear for 2 minutes on each side.
- Introduce the pan in the oven and bake the fish at 425 degrees F for 7 minutes.
- Meanwhile, in a bowl, mix the quinoa with the remaining ingredients, toss and divide between plates.
- Add the fish next to the quinoa mix and serve right away.

Nutrition:

calories 364, fat 15.4, fiber 11.2, carbs 56.4, protein 24.5

Orange-spiced Pumpkin Hummus

Servings:4

Cooking Time:5 Minutes

Ingredients:

- 1 tbsp. maple syrup
- 1/2 tsp. salt
- 1 can (16 oz.) garbanzo beans
- 1/8 tsp. ginger or nutmeg
- 1 cup canned pumpkin Blend,
- 1/8 tsp. cinnamon
- 1/4 cup tahini
- 1 tbsp. fresh orange juice
- Pinch of orange zest, for garnish
- 1 tbsp. apple cider vinegar

Directions:

- Mix all the ingredients in a food processor or blender until slightly chunky.
- Serve right away, and enjoy!

Nutrition:

Calories: 291 ,Fats: 22.9 g ,Carbs: 15 g ,Protein: 12 g

Artichoke Skewers

Servings:4

Cooking Time:10 Minutes

Ingredients:

- 4 prosciutto slices
- 4 artichoke hearts, canned
- 4 kalamata olives
- 4 cherry tomatoes
- ¼ teaspoon cayenne pepper
- ¼ teaspoon sunflower oil

Directions:

- Skewer prosciutto slices, artichoke hearts, kalamata olives, and cherry tomatoes on the wooden skewers.
- Sprinkle antipasto skewers with sunflower oil and cayenne pepper.

Nutrition:

calories 152, fat 3.7, fiber 10.8, carbs 23.2, protein 11.1

Honey Balsamic Salmon

Servings:2

Cooking Time:3 Minutes

Ingredients:

- 2 salmon fillets
- 1/4 tsp red pepper flakes
- 2 tbsp honey
- 2 tbsp balsamic vinegar
- 1 cup of water
- Pepper
- Salt

Directions:

- Pour water into the instant pot and place trivet in the pot.
- In a small bowl, mix together honey, red pepper flakes, and vinegar.
- Brush fish fillets with honey mixture and place on top of the trivet.
- Seal pot with lid and cook on high for 3 minutes.
- Once done, release pressure using quick release. Remove lid.
- Serve and enjoy.

Nutrition:

Calories 303 Fat 11 g Carbohydrates 17.6 g Sugar 17.3 g Protein 34.6 g Cholesterol 78 mg

www.ingramcontent.com/pod-product-compliance
Lightning Source LLC
Chambersburg PA
CBHW050231120526
44590CB00016B/2045